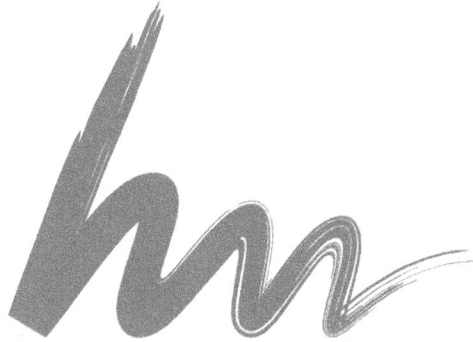

harmonic movement™

BRIAN JAMES KROEKER

PUBLISHED BY BURNING HEART STUDIO
VICTORIA, CANADA

**When you move with your breath,
you move to the rhythm of life.**

Book Design by Brian James Kroeker
Photographs by Debra Stapleton

Second Edition, June 2016
Third Edition, January 2018

More information: www.burningheartyoga.com

contents

ACKNOWLEDGMENTS

Infinite love and gratitude to my wife Debbie, who many years ago inspired me to live to my full potential, and has unfailingly supported me every step of the way.

I extend gratitude to all my teachers and their teachers, especially Sri T. Krishnamacharya and TKV Desikachar for all they have done to make the techniques of the great yoga tradition accessible and relevant to modern people, regardless of age, body type, gender or cultural background. I hope that my efforts honour their work.

And to my parents, who gave me the gift of this beautiful life. I wouldn't be here without you.

Brian James Kroeker
January 2016

When you become one with your breath, you can become one with anything.

introduction

There is a vast, great intelligence at work in you, right now, at this very moment.

Before you humbly scoff, just pause for a moment, close your eyes and notice your breath. See how it continues giving you life even when you aren't thinking about it? Take note of the incredible design of your body: the organs, muscles, fluids and bones all functioning harmoniously to keep you alive. Now listen to the rhythm of your heartbeat, providing the constant pulse of life throughout your entire body, sending blood to the brain that we often consider to be the isolated abode of wisdom and intelligence.

The truth is that your *whole body* is a great and wondrous intelligence at work — the same intelligence that tells an acorn how to grow into an oak tree; that tells a baby bird when it's time to emerge from its egg, or an apple to drop from its branch. It sets the rhythm of the tides, the spin of the earth. It's the timeless power and intelligence behind the infinite cosmic cycles of life, death and rebirth that we call Nature, Life or God.

You see, *you are* that great power, intelligence and wonder. The practices in this workbook are designed to awaken you to that power, to show you how you can quiet your mind and listen to the intelligence of your body; to remind you that *you are a natural wonder.*

Harmonize Your Mind, Breath & Body

Have you ever tried to sleep but your mind just won't settle down? Tried to focus but your thoughts keep jumping from one thing to another? We've all had the experience of lying in bed, mentally exhausted but experiencing a feeling of restlessness in our body. Have you ever attempted to just sit and think of nothing? It's not easy... some would even say impossible.

During our usual day-to-day activities, our body and mind are often functioning at completely different frequencies, producing a dissonance that we experience as distraction, mental fog, and feelings of stress, tension and general anxiety. This disharmony can be as uncomfortable as listening to an orchestra tuning up before a concert. Harmonic Movement combines breathwork and functional, natural movement in a powerful practice that effectively and effortlessly brings your mind and body into total harmony.

5 Elements of Harmonic Movement

01 Rhythm
Your breath is the rhythm of life and the key to Harmonic Movement. The first step is learning how to regulate your breath rhythm.

02 Tempo
Your breath rhythm establishes the tempo for your practice. Sometimes you might want a relaxed and downtempo practice, other times a more energetic and uptempo practice. You can adjust the tempo of your practice to complement or shift your energy levels.

03 Harmony

When you synchronize a movement to the rhythm of your breath it brings body and mind into total harmony. When body and mind are in harmony, it creates a calm, focused and joyful state.

04 Flow

A flow is a movement loop that you can seamlessly repeat over and over. As you cycle through the flow it turns into a moving meditation and breath and body become one.

05 Rest

Movement allows for stillness. The pauses between your inhalation and exhalation become brief moments of stillness in your movement. Every practice ends with a period of rest and reflection.

The harmony of mind, breath and body induces a state of alertness, relaxation, focus, and clarity known as "flow". The flow state has been known to yogis, musicians, martial artists and meditators for thousands of years and recent research has shown that it enhances learning, athletic performance, work productivity, creativity and increases feelings of happiness, joy and general well-being.

Feeling is Knowing

The simple but powerful method that I present step-by-step in this book is a distillation of over twenty years of practice and study of the mind and body traditions of many cultures, including hatha yoga, western fitness, global shamanic traditions, and various martial arts. While I could write for pages about the positive benefits that I've experienced through my years of daily practice, I'd rather have you discover them for yourself. I'm confident that if you follow the instructions in this workbook, you'll feel the effects for yourself immediately. After all, *feeling is knowing!*

free your breath and your mind will follow.

Keep it Simple. Stay Consistent.

3 Tips for Developing a Daily Practice

01 Timing
Try to practice at the same time every day, preferably first thing in the morning before you check your email or turn on your phone — it's a time when you're the least distracted and most able to focus on your practice.

02 Simplicity
Even if you think you could easily add an hour-long practice session to your daily routine, stick to just 10-20 minutes for the first month. If you find you have extra time to do another practice, do it in the evening to unwind and de-stress from your day.

03 Consistency
Make a promise to yourself to practice every day for at least a month. Set your phone to send you reminders every evening before bed, and mark your calendar when you're done every morning. It helps to have someone or something to be accountable to, even if it's just your calendar!

To experience increasing benefits over the long-term, keep your practice simple and stay consistent. Start with a 10- to 20-minute practice every morning for the first thirty days, then build on it. There are some sample sequences and complete practices at the end of the book to get you started.

Most importantly, have fun and be creative! If you're not enjoying your practice you won't continue to do it. Experiment with your own Harmonic Movement sequences and *find your own flow* — allow your curiosity to guide you. Explore movement practices like Qi Gong and Tai Chi, yoga, dance, martial arts — even physiotherapy — and apply the breathing techniques you'll learn in this book to transform them into a moving meditation. I've provided some blank pages in the back so you can record your own sequences and movements that you learn from other sources.

Enjoy your breath, enjoy your life.

1.0 breathe

Your breath is the key to experiencing total mind and body harmony.

When you combine the breathing technique described in the next few pages with mindful movement, you're able to harmonize your body and mind quickly and effortlessly. *Harmonic Movement begins with your breath.*

Once you learn the fundamental technique of regulating your breath with a gentle constriction of your throat — sometimes called *ocean breath* because of the wave-like sound it produces — you're able to tap into your nervous system and calm your mind, slow your heart rate, reduce stress and even improve your digestion.

Master this technique and you'll have an effective and reliable tool that you can call on whenever you need to calm down and focus.

exercise 1.1

ocean breath

Set aside 5-10 minutes to try this first exercise.
Find a quiet place where you won't be disturbed or feel self-conscious. The acoustics in your bathroom can help you listen to, and fine tune your breath.

"AHH"

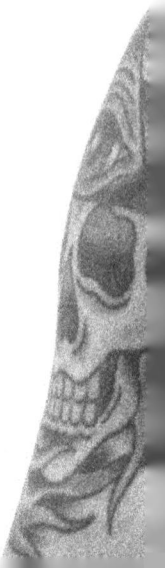

01 Breath with sound.
Inhale through your mouth
making an *ahh* sound like
you've just seen a triple
rainbow or a beautiful sunset.

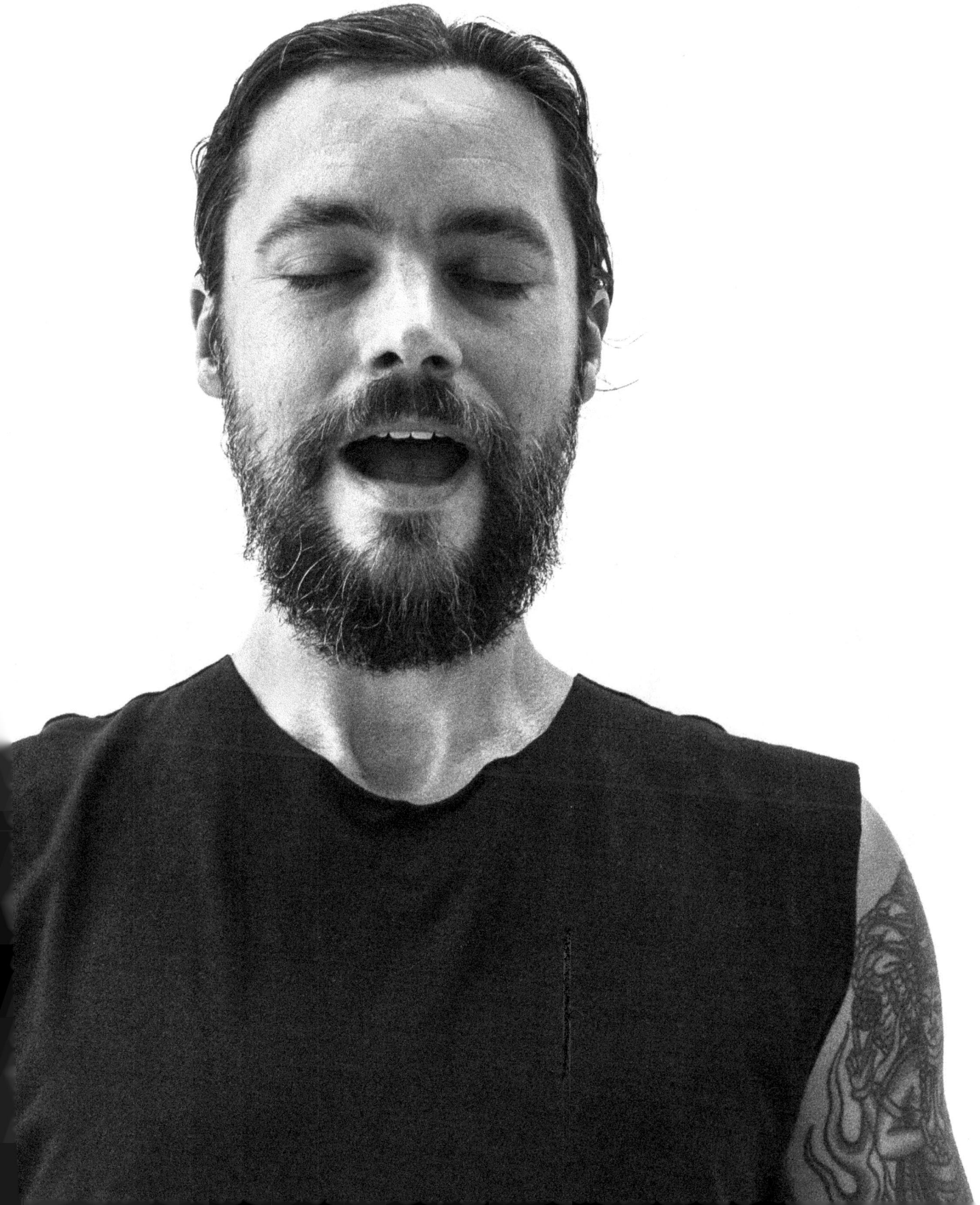

02 Exhale out your mouth making a *haa* sound. Pretend that you're fogging your sunglasses like you're going to clean them. *Ah-ha!* Now you've got it!

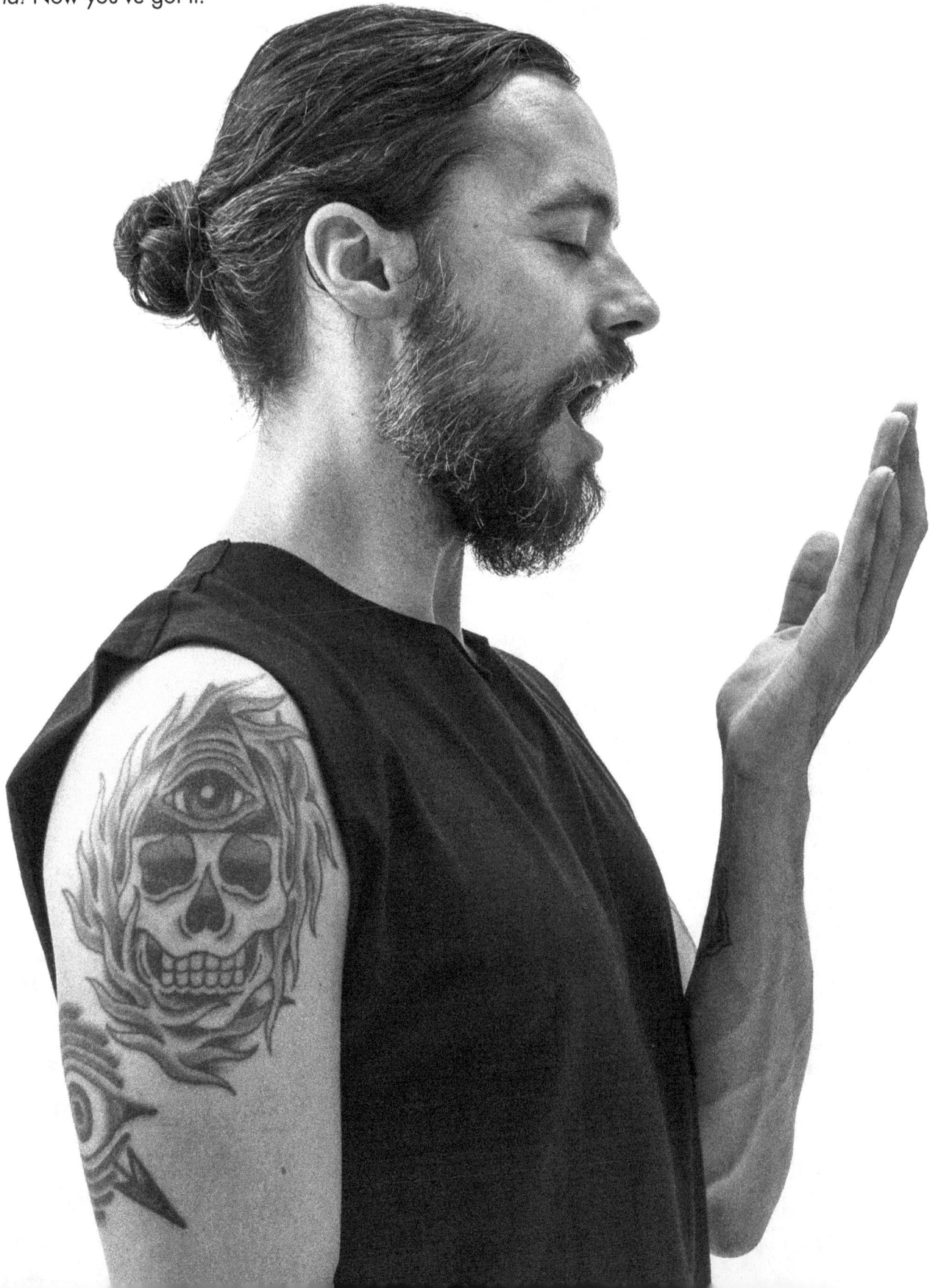

"HAA"

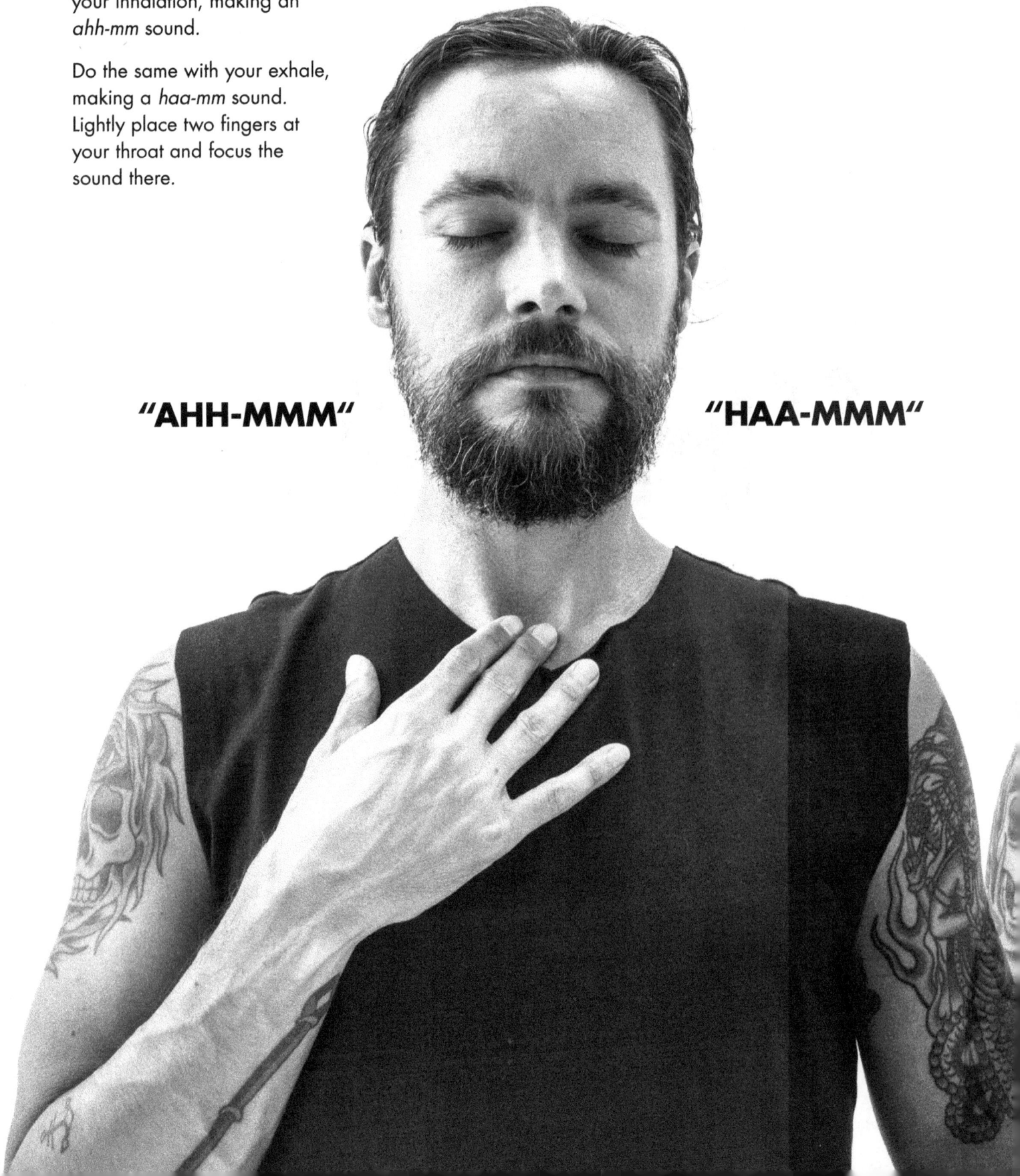

03 Focus the sound.

When you're comfortable making the sound on both the inhale and exhale, try closing your mouth midway through your inhalation, making an *ahh-mm* sound.

Do the same with your exhale, making a *haa-mm* sound. Lightly place two fingers at your throat and focus the sound there.

"AHH-MMM"

"HAA-MMM"

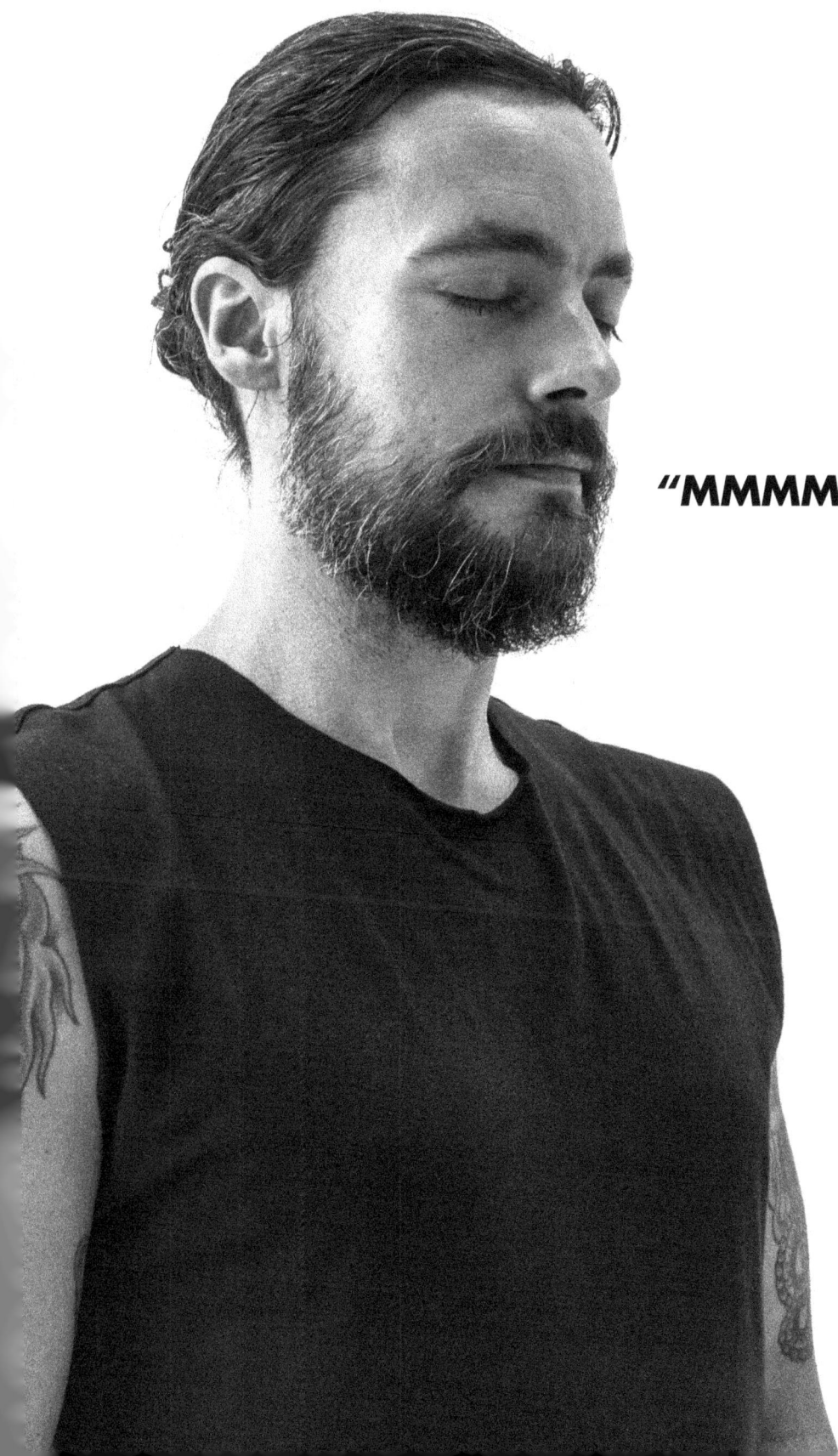

04 Ocean breath.

Now try a full inhale and exhale with your lips sealed and jaw relaxed, creating a sound chamber for your breath. The sound resembles ocean waves, ebbing and flowing, in and out.

Try placing the tip of your tongue on the roof of your mouth, this will help keep your jaw relaxed and the inside of your mouth open and resonant. You might feel your breath swirling around at the back of your throat.

"MMMMM"

Before moving on...

Take some time getting comfortable at this stage before moving on, it's the key to the whole practice.

05 Breath awareness.

Begin your inhalation by breathing into your chest first. As your inhalation deepens, allow your belly to expand.

As you inhale, your diaphragm — the double-domed muscle separating your chest and abdominal cavities — contracts and moves downward, creating space in your lungs for air to enter. It's this volume change in your chest that causes your belly to expand.

Visualize this internal movement as you feel it happening with your hands.

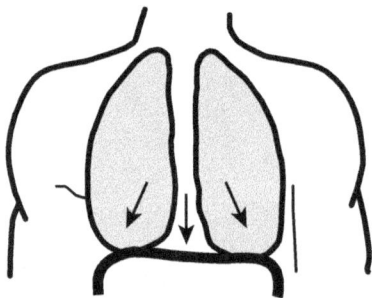

fig 01. Diaphragm on inhale
(contracted position)

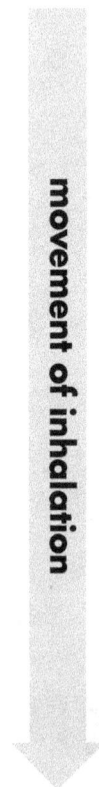

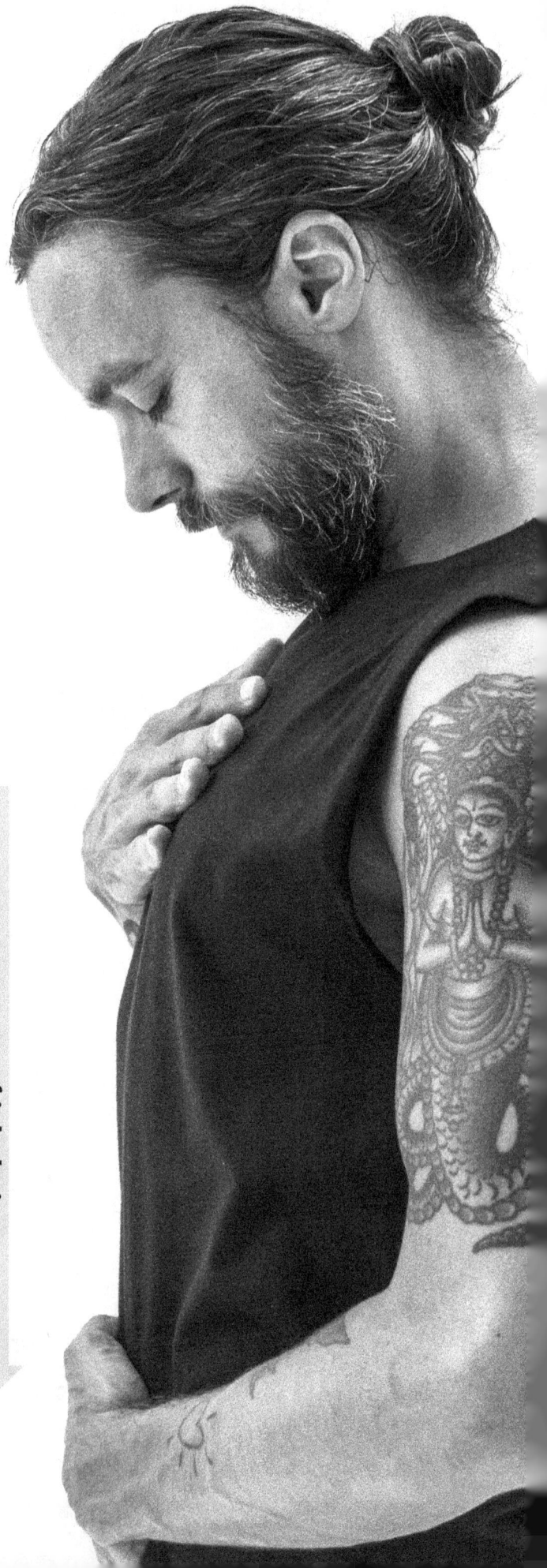

movement of inhalation

06 Begin your exhalation by contracting your lower abdominals first. As the air leaves your lungs feel your chest relax second.

Just as you inhaled from the top down, your exhalation happens in a bottom up sequence. Your chest is the point of awareness on inhale; your lower abdominals the point of awareness on exhale.

As you exhale, visualize your diaphragm returning to it's domed at-rest shape.

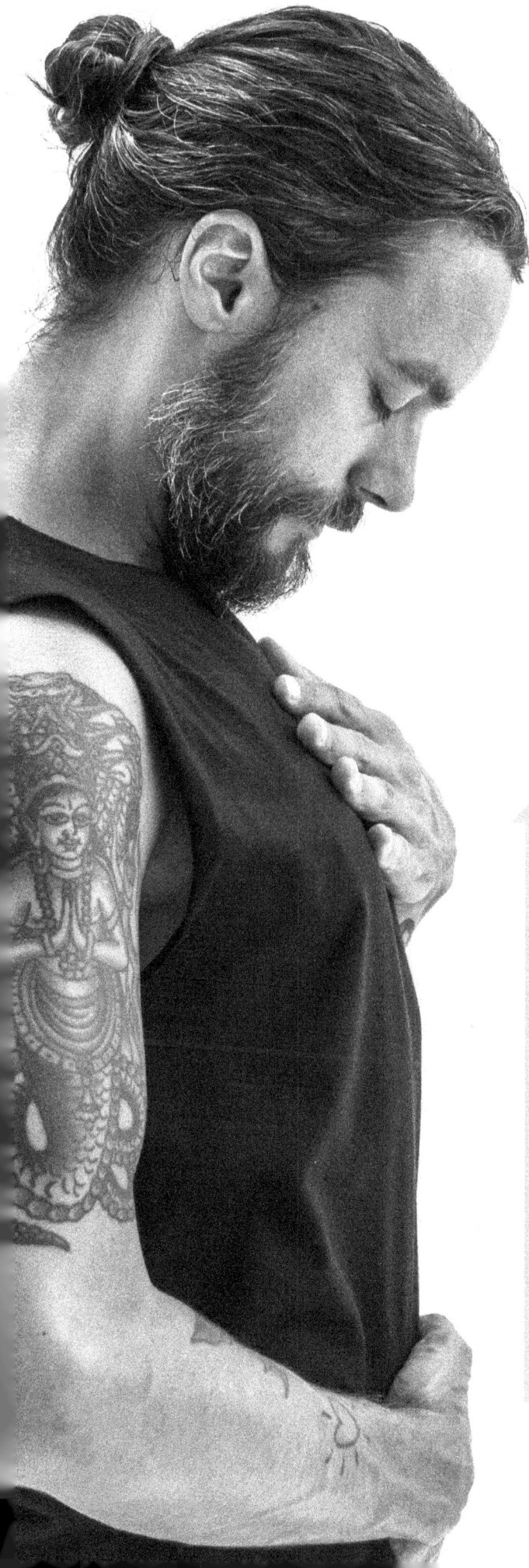

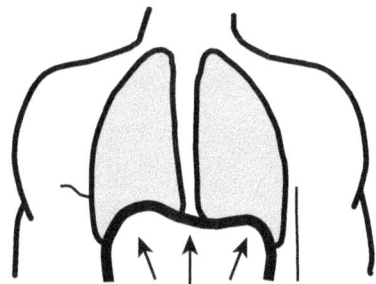

movement of exhalation

fig 02. Diaphragm on exhale
(relaxed position)

07 Breath rhythm.

Focus on maintaining a steady breath rhythm, making the inhalation and exhalation an equal length. It may help to silently count along, just like a musician or dancer keeping time. Make your breath as long and smooth as you comfortably can without struggling.

Often, when first attempting to regulate our breathing, we find that one part of our breath is naturally longer than the other. Over time, with consistent practice, your inhale and exhale will become equally strong, smooth and comfortable.

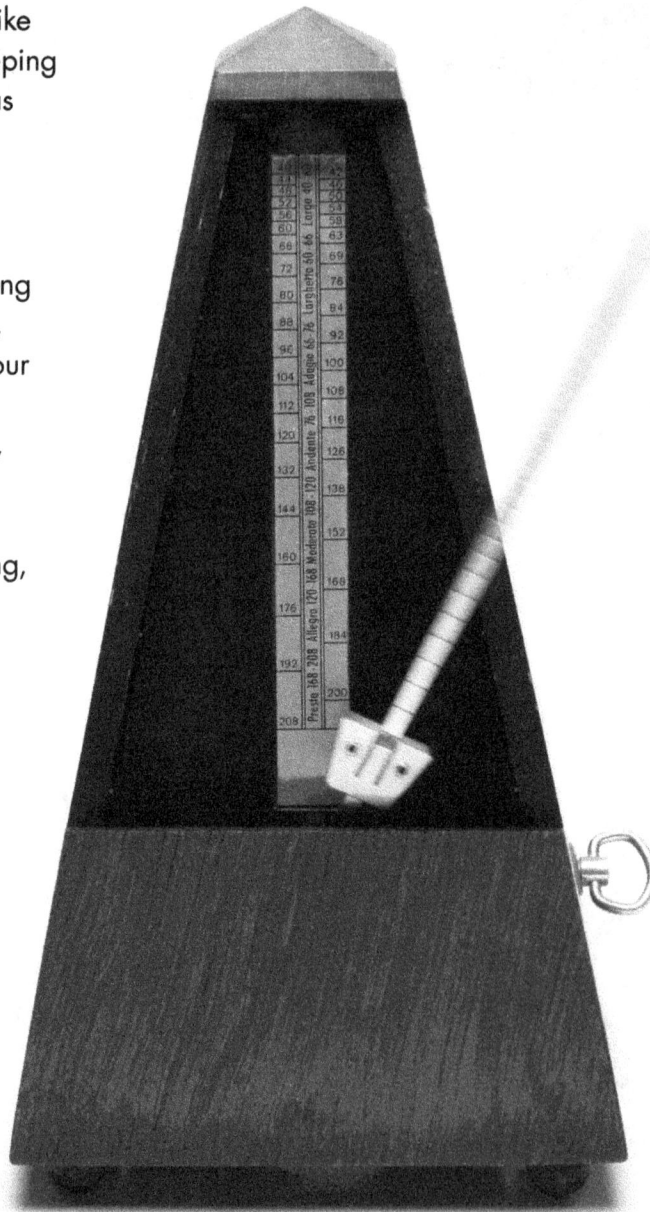

"inhale, 2, 3, 4...
exhale, 2, 3, 4..."

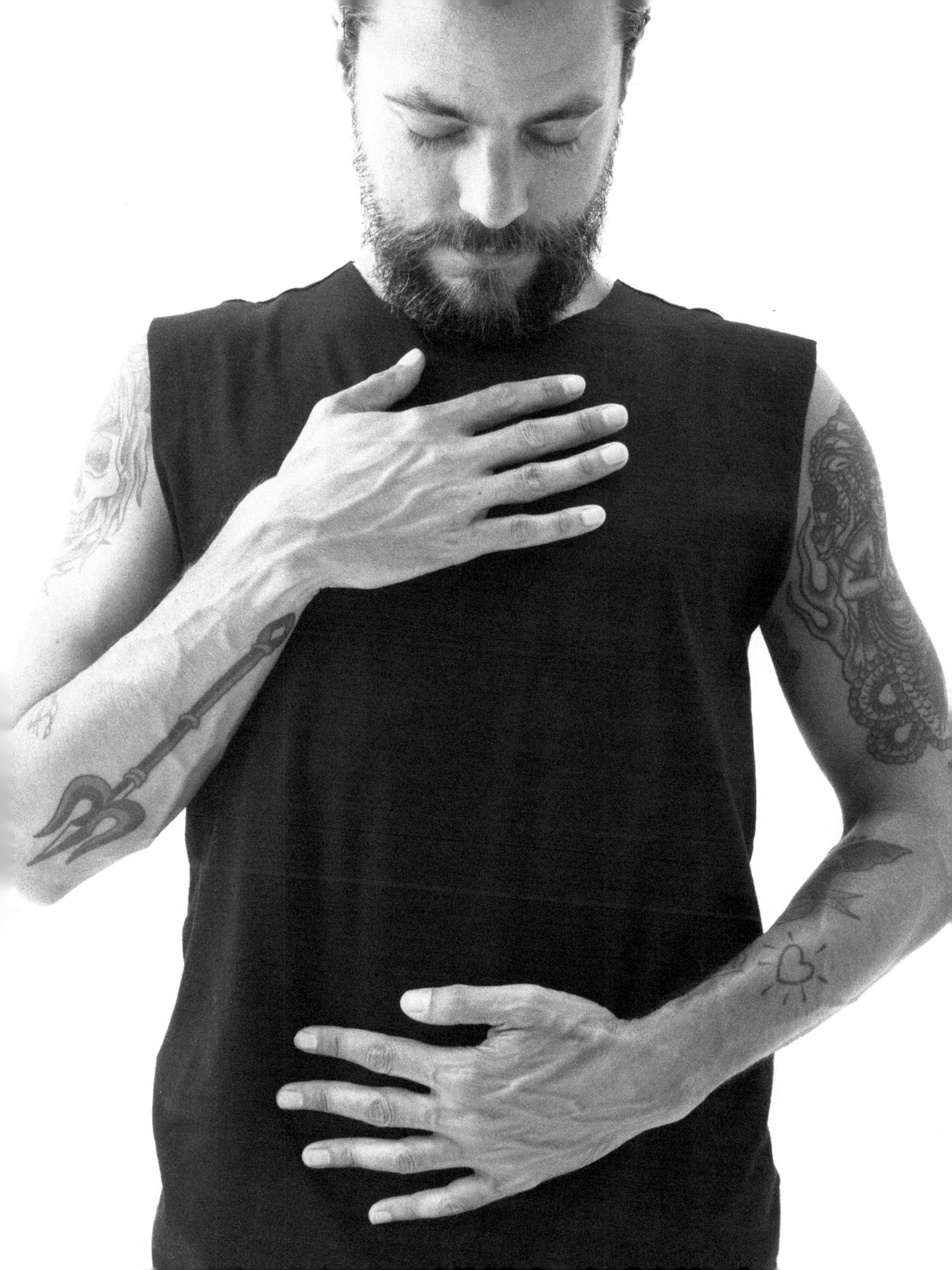

2.0 harmonize

The next step is to harmonize your body and breath.

We do this by synchronizing your body movement with the steady rhythmic movement of your breath. Once body-breath harmony is established in simple isolated movements, we can start to introduce more dynamism and complexity, forming integrated movement chains by linking movements together to create flow.

Be sure to practice the two exercises in this chapter before moving on to the more complex movements presented later in the book.
Spend some time really exploring the connection between your breath and body movement.
Try to approach these exercises with a quality of "no mind" — let go of any pre-conceived ideas of how the movements should *look*, and focus on how they *feel*. Let your movement become a pure expression of your breath, let your breath become your teacher, your *guru*.

surf your breath.

exercise 2.1

riding the wave of your breath

This is a movement exercise that allows us to experience our breath as a wave-like motion in our body, expanding and contracting.

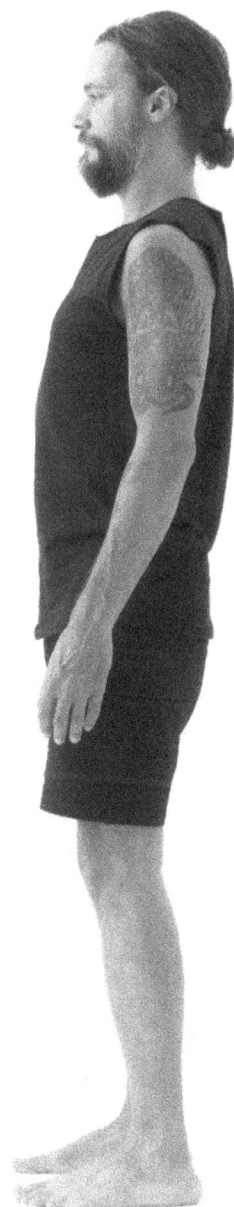

01 Begin standing.
Stand with your feet parallel and hip width, arms relaxed at your side, knees slightly bent, spine tall, chest open, gaze toward the horizon.

02 Regulate your breath.
Establish a steady, even breath for a few rounds, as described in the previous section. Focus on making the sound smooth and relaxed.

inhale

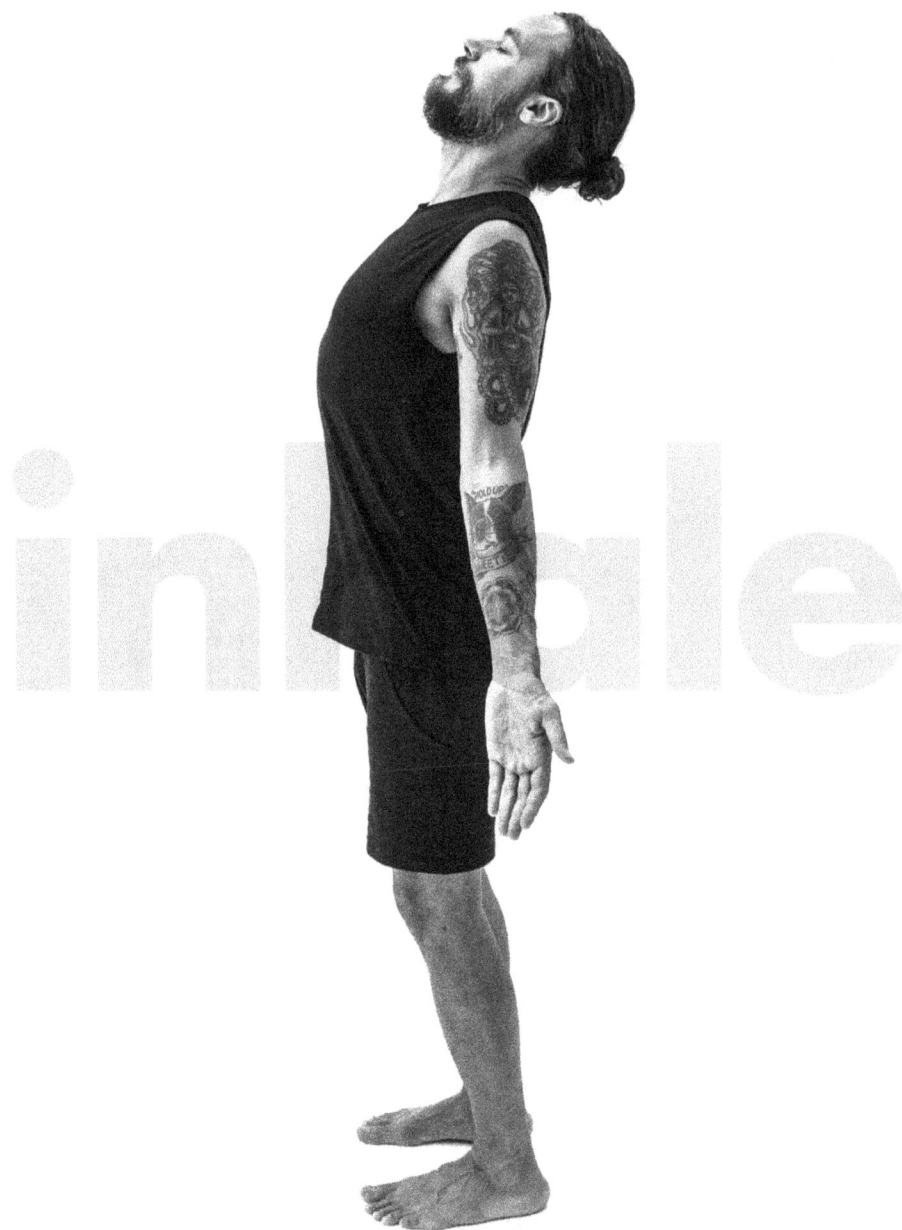

03 Inhale is expansion.

As you inhale, lift your head and chest, and roll your shoulders back. Let your arms and hands spiral open. Feel as though you are expanding and opening outward from the center of your chest. As you increase the back arch, engage the muscles in your backside for support. Go only as deeply as you feel comfortable.

exhale

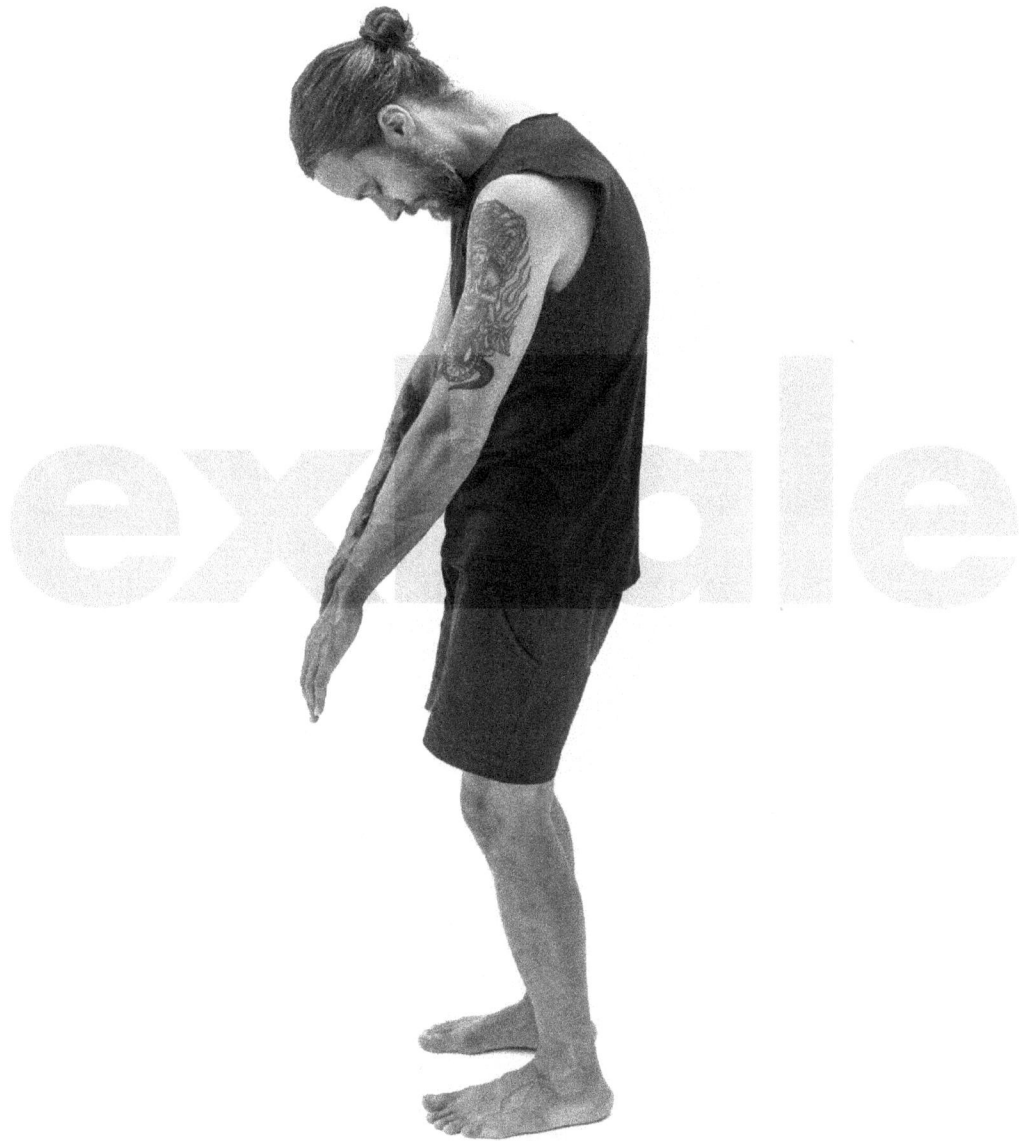

04 Exhale is contraction.

Begin your exhalation by first contracting your abdominals. Allow your shoulders and arms to roll forward, dropping your chin and slightly bending your knees. As you complete your exhale, visualize yourself drawing in toward your physical center, just below your navel. Repeat the movement a number of times until you have the feeling of breath and body becoming one.

inhale is receiving

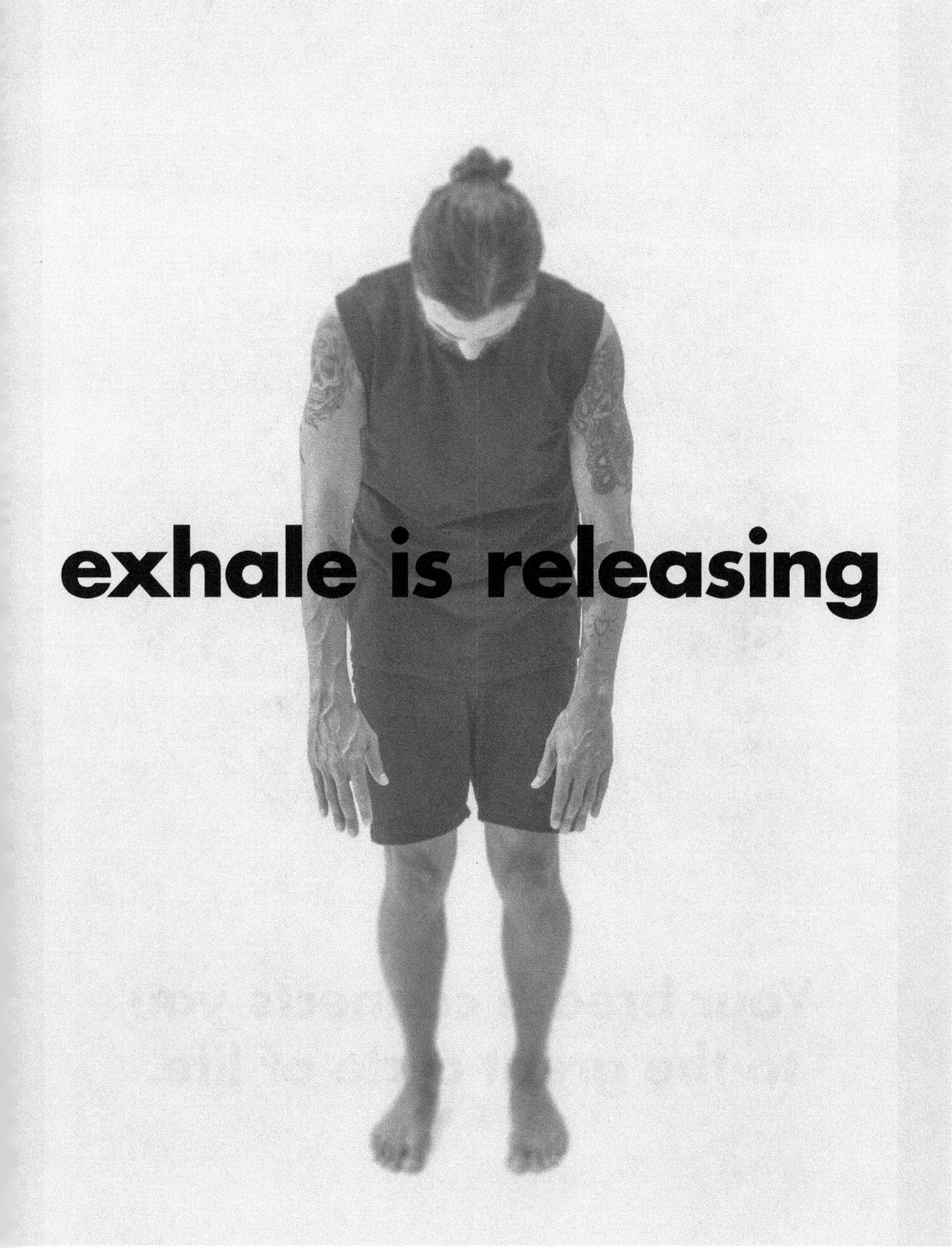

exhale is releasing

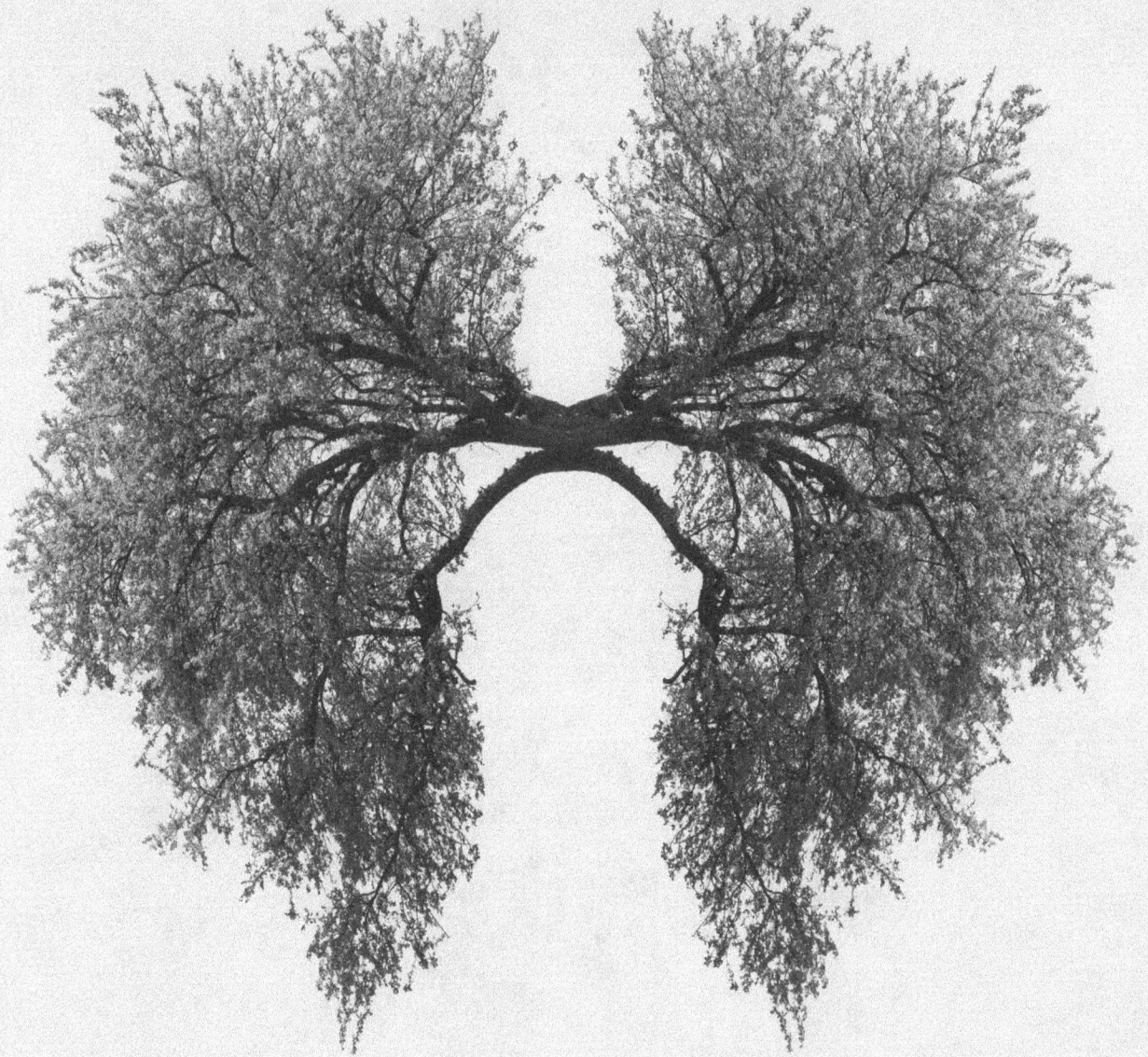

Your breath connects you to the great cycle of life.

enveloping the movement

This exercise helps us to refine the relationship between our breath and body as we start to envelop each movement with our breath.

01 Begin standing.
Stand with your feet parallel and hip width, arms relaxed at your side, knees slightly bent, spine tall, chest open, gazing toward the horizon.

02 Regulate your breath.
Establish a steady, even breath for a few rounds, as described in the previous section. Focus on making the sound smooth and relaxed.

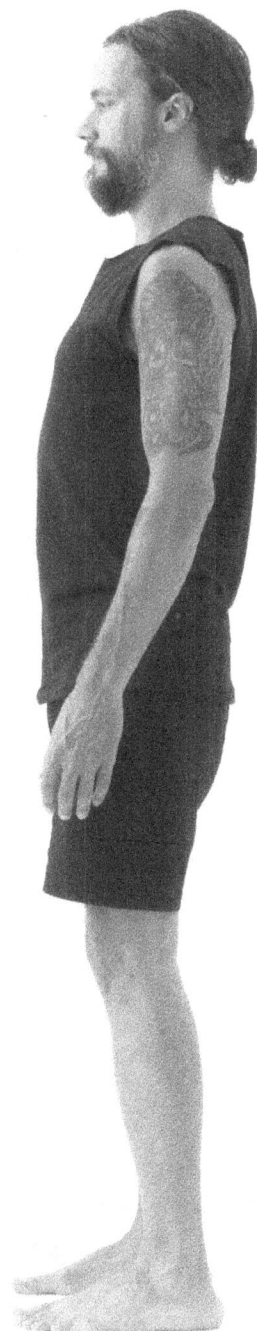

exercise 2.2
enveloping the movement

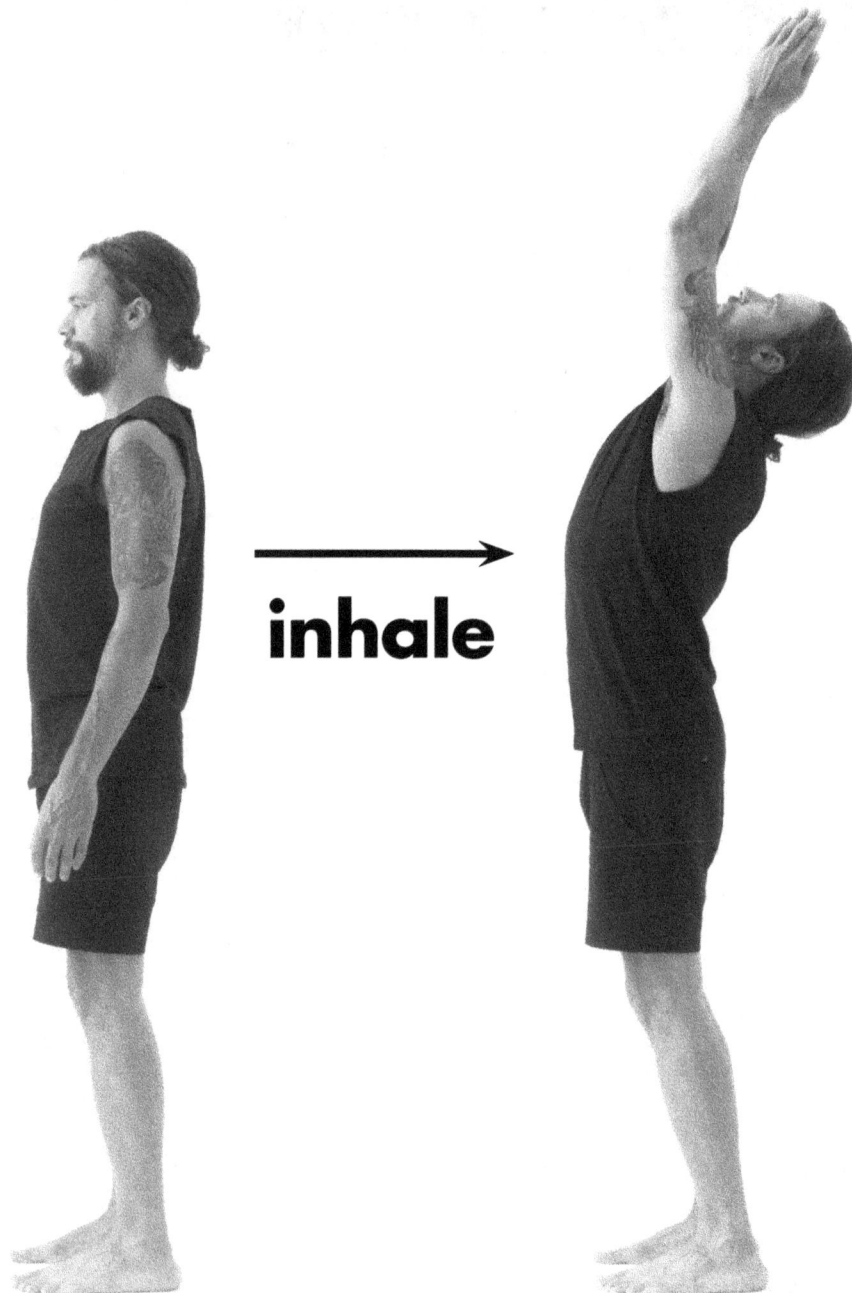

inhale

03 Inhale arms up.

Inhale and sweep your arms out from your sides and overhead in a circular motion. Look up and see your hands come together just before your inhalation is complete.

exhale

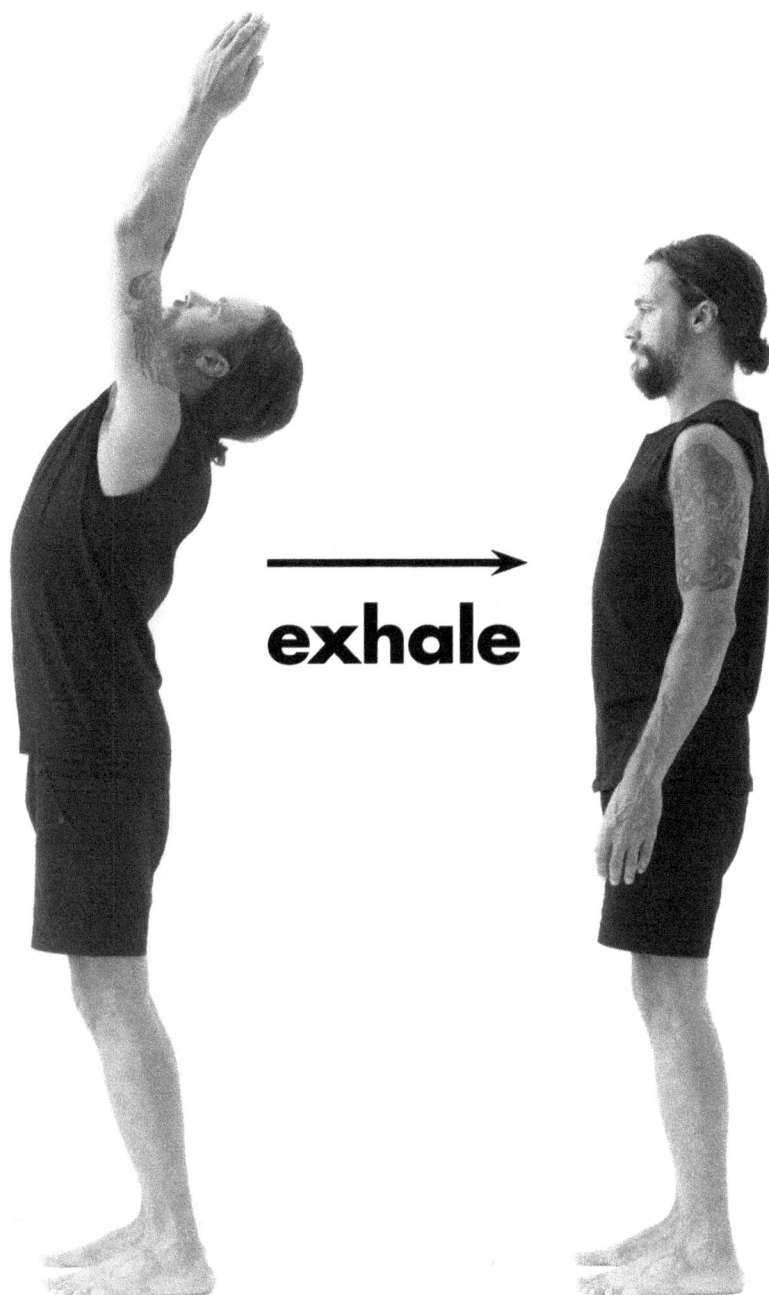

04 Exhale arms down.
Exhale and return your arms to your side and gaze to the horizon, finishing the movement
slightly before your exhalation is complete.

breath

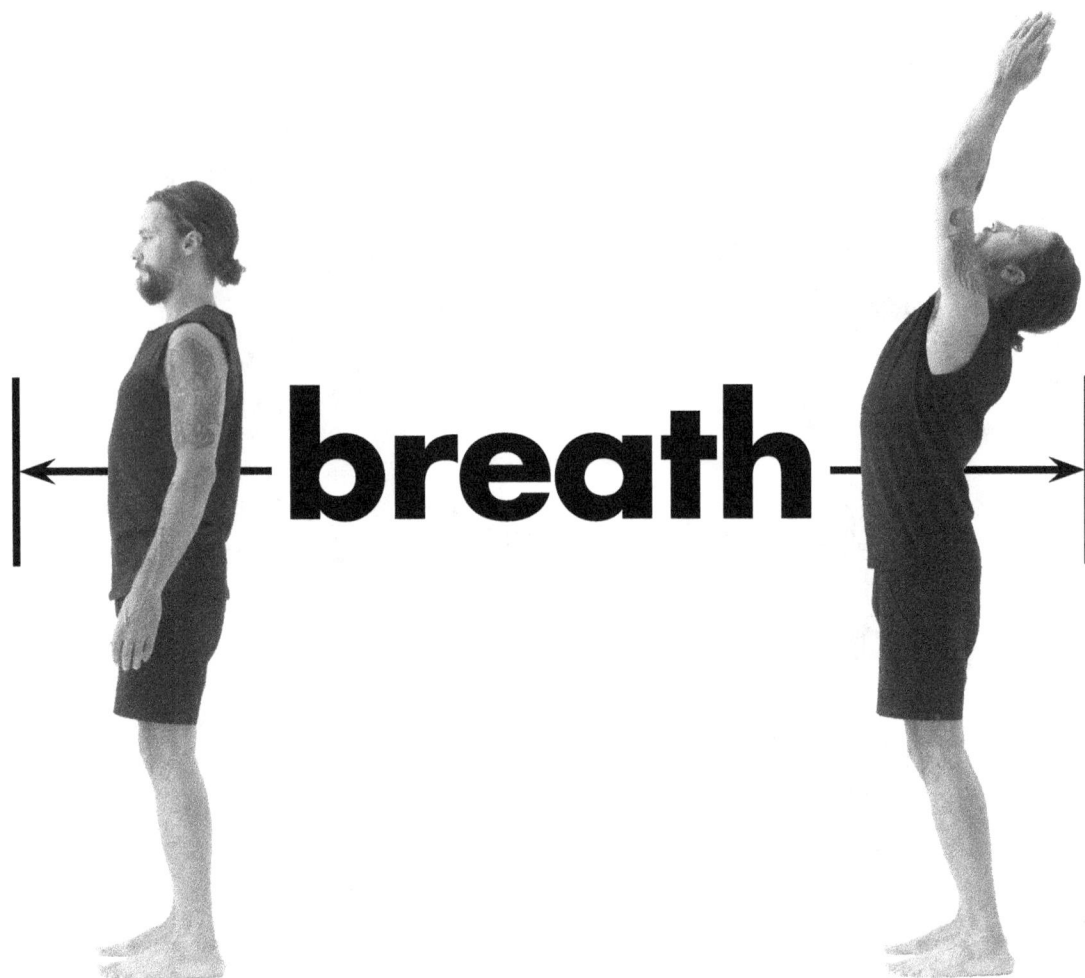

Breath is longer than movement.

05 Continue raising and lowering your arms with the inhalation and exhalation, focusing on making your breath slightly longer than your movements. Allow your breath to envelop the movement. Just like the drummer in a band, your breath sets the tempo of your practice, and maintains a steady rhythm throughout. Every movement follows the cue of your breath.

1
inhale

2
pause

3
exhale

4
pause

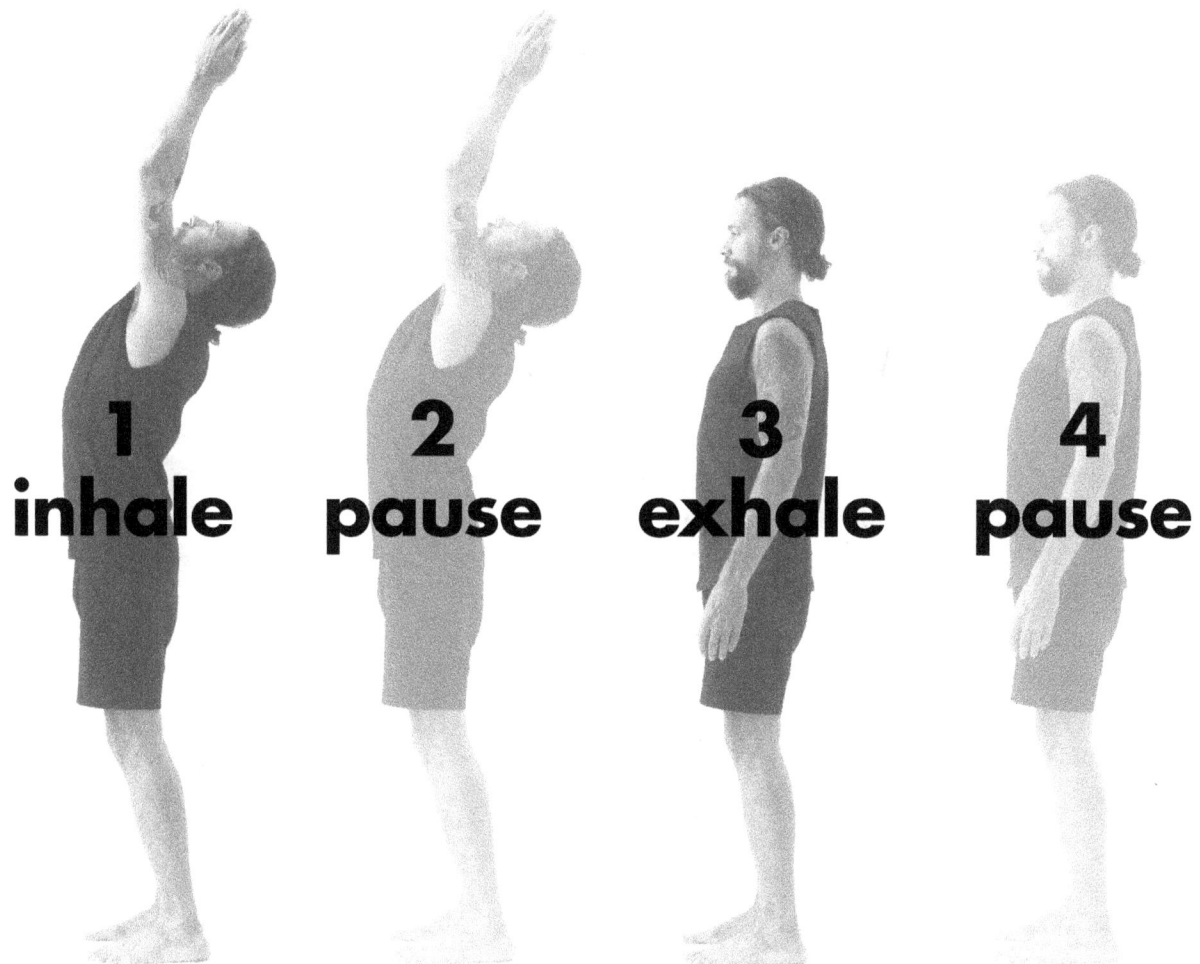

There are four parts to every breath.

06 In the natural pauses between your inhale and exhale, allow for moments of stillness in your body and mind. As you get comfortable syncing your breath and movement, you can explore lengthening these pauses. There's power in the pause!

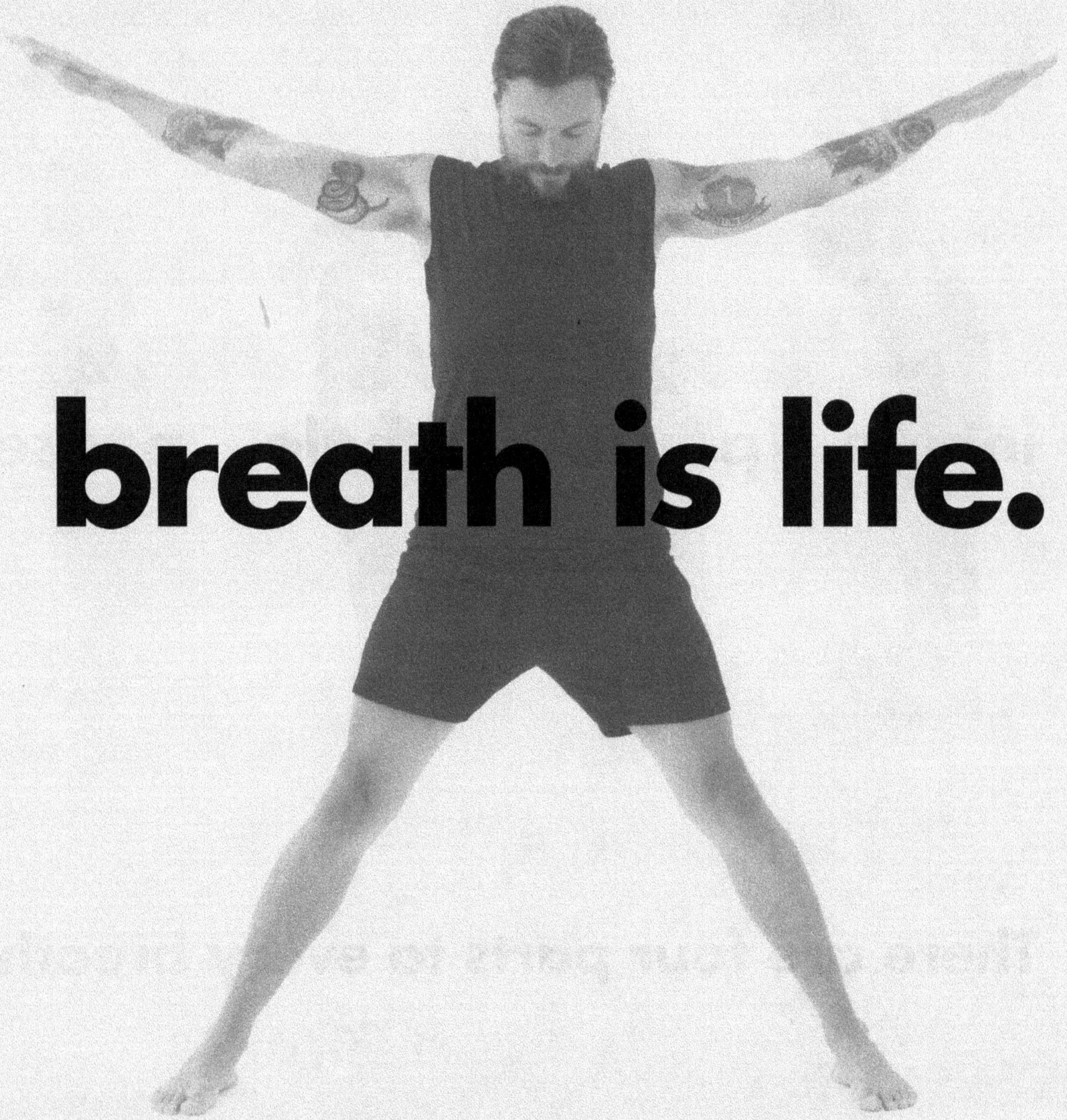

breath is life.

move with life.

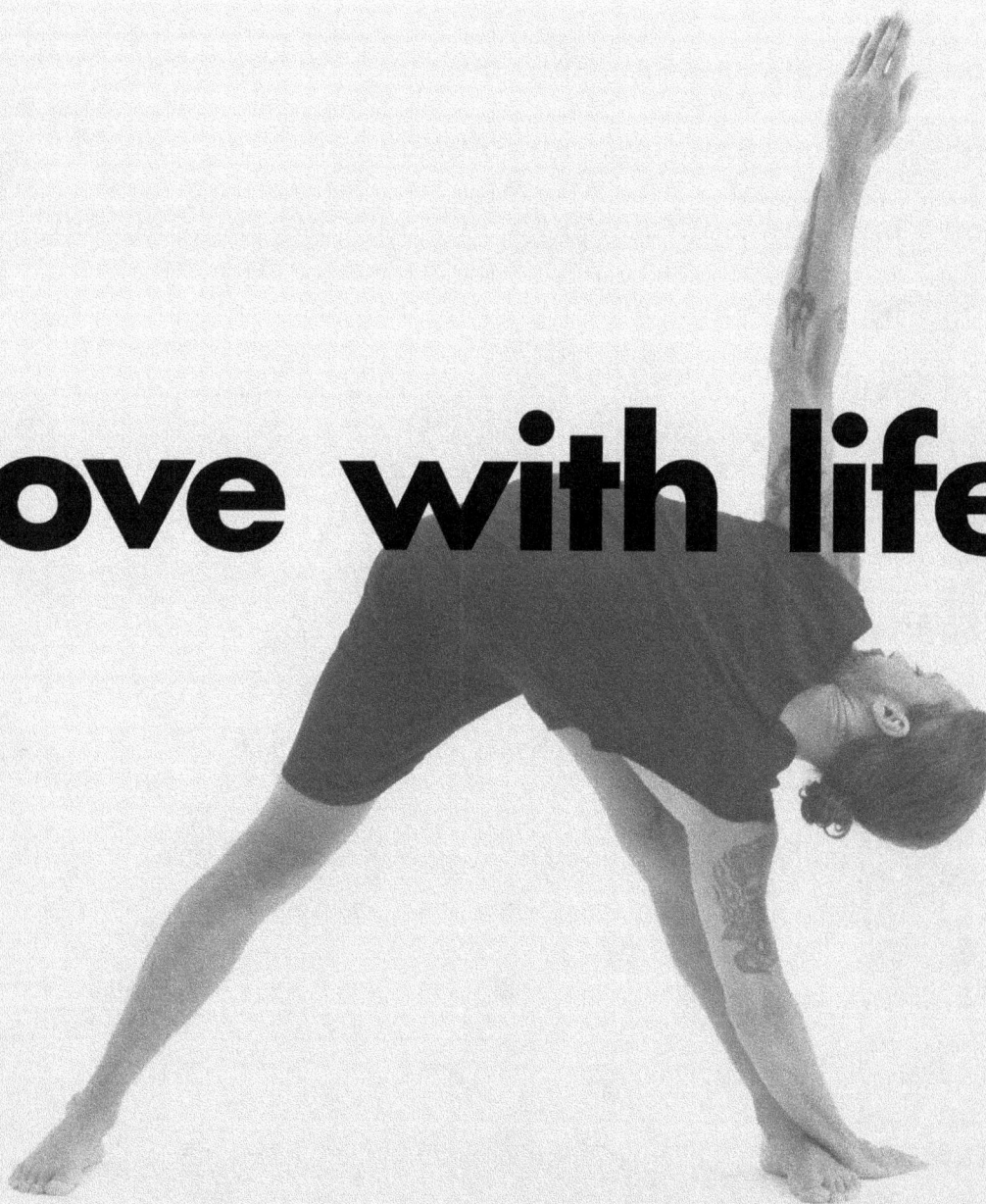

3.0 move

You can apply the Harmonic Movement method to a vast array of natural human movements.

Start by exploring the movements on the following pages to develop your own "movement toolbox" based on your individual physical needs and unique interests. Once you are comfortable with the method, you can apply it to just about any two-stage movement pattern, transforming it into a powerful moving meditation.

On the following pages there are a number of isolated movements to get you started and some examples of integrated "flows" that link movements together in a chain that can be seamlessly repeated. At first, try the isolated movements in the order they're presented for five or more cycles of breath. Once they're familiar to you, use them to design your own practice sequences.

Let these examples act as a starting point for our practice. Be creative, explore, and *find your own flow*.

Find Your Own Flow: Some Tips
For Developing a Personal Practice

Stay curious, be creative and look for inspiration in many places. There are an infinite amount of movement patterns that you can enhance by applying the Harmonic Movement technique. I encourage you to experiment with the sequences in this book and then develop your own (there's room in the back to record what you learn). The internet, library and nature are great places to start your research.

Let your practice be a catalyst for learning. The movements I've included here are inspired by hatha yoga, Indian wrestling exercises, calisthenics, gymnastics, Pilates, martial arts and natural human and animal movement patterns. There's a vast body of knowledge to draw from, both ancient and modern.

Let your movement practice be a way to connect. Seek out experts and other movement enthusiasts. Observe other movers, and observe your own patterns. Start a movement journal. Create or find a community of movers — we learn best with friends. Share what you discover and inspire others to get out and move!

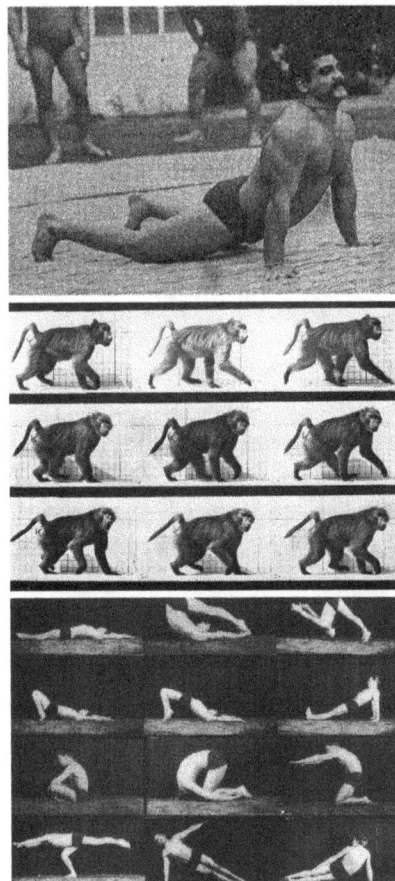

From top to bottom:
Indian wrestler performing a Hindu pushup; Edward Muybridge study of baboon movement; Muybridge's study of Joseph Pilates' movement.

4 Easy Steps to Total Mind & Body Harmony

As you explore applying the Harmonic Movement method to sequences found in and outside this book, remember these basic steps to harmonize your body, breath and mind (in that order). In just a short time, this method will become second nature and you soon may find yourself applying it to movements automatically.

1. REGULATE YOUR BREATH. Make it steady, even and constant. Your breath is the key to extablishing mind and body harmony.

2. SYNCHRONIZE BODY AND BREATH MOVEMENT. Your body movements follow your breath. Your breath should be slightly longer than the movement — remember, your breath envelops your movement.

3. INHALATION IS EXPANDING. Inhalation accompanies expansive, lengthening movements and limbs moving away from your center, which creates space for the incoming breath.

4. EXHALATION IS CONTRACTING. Exhalation accompanies contracting movements and limbs moving into your center, helping to express the breath completely.

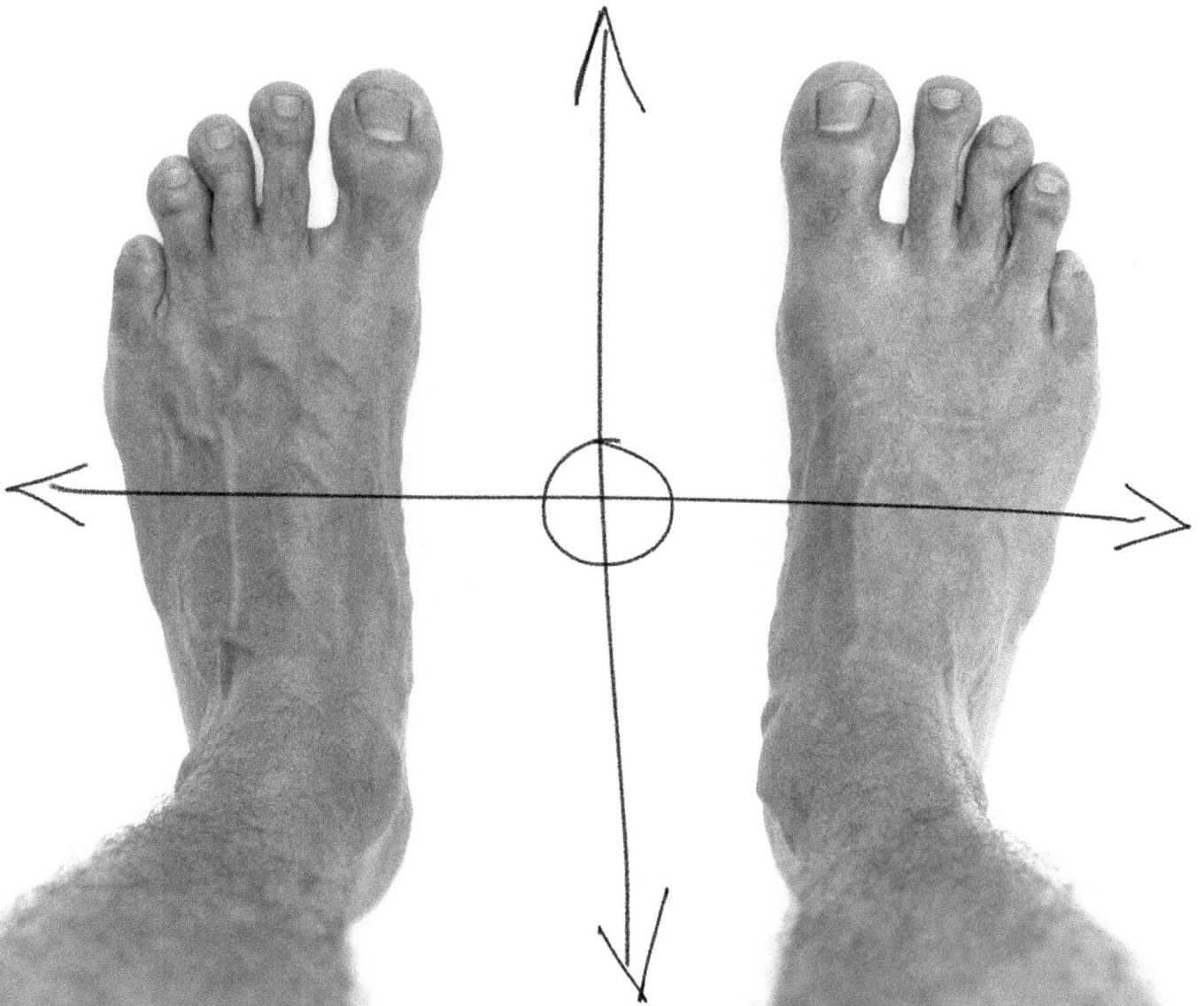

EQUAL STANDING

establish your foundation.

Firmly connect to the earth with equal weight in both feet, front to back, left to right.

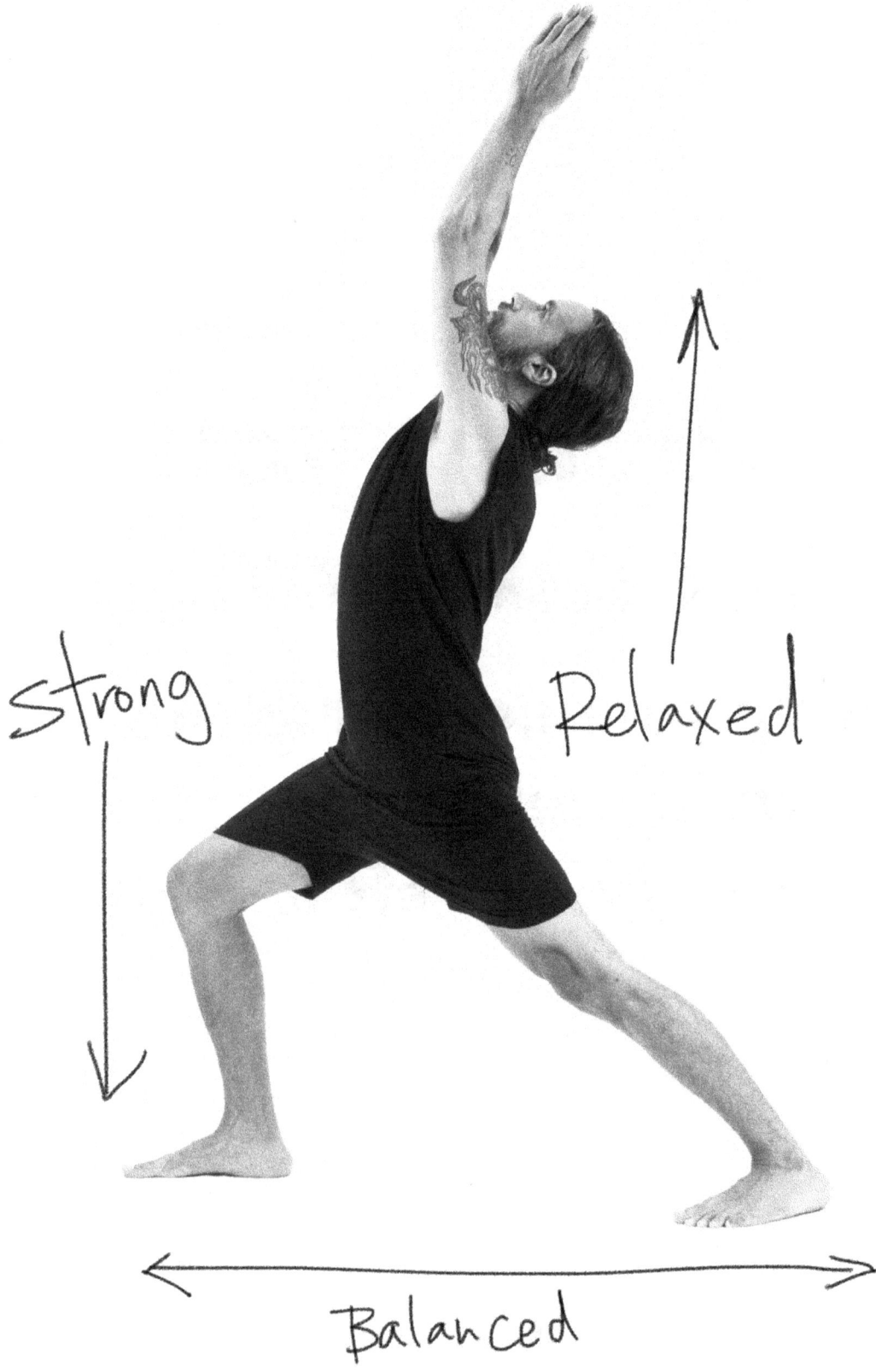

Strong

Relaxed

Balanced

GENERAL TIP FOR STANDING MOVEMENTS #2

be equally strong and relaxed.

Be strong where you need to, and soft where you can.

3.1 standing movements

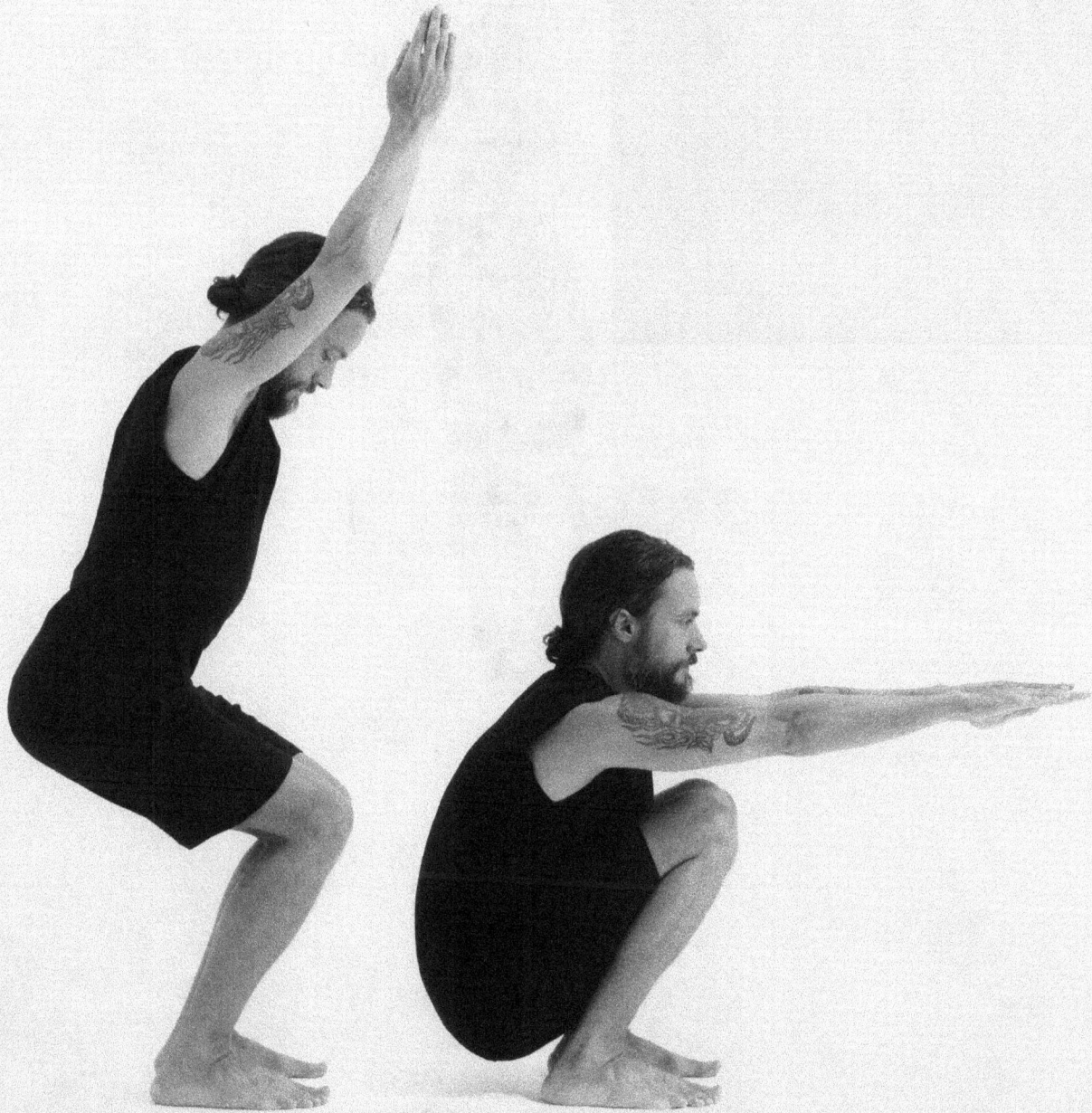

equal standing posture

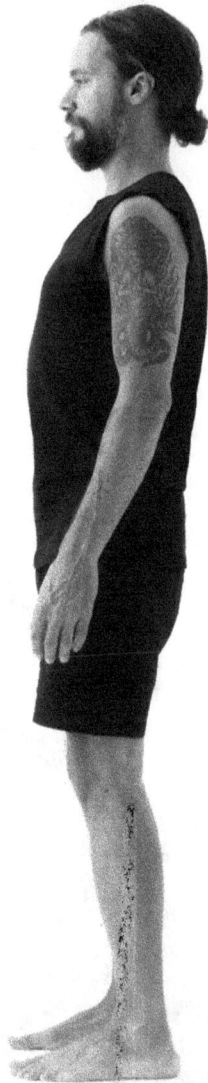

Start in the equal standing posture where your feet are parallel and hip width with equal weight from toes to heels. Arrange the rest of your body around the centerline that runs from the crown of your head to the center of the earth. Your posture should be both alert and relaxed at the same time.

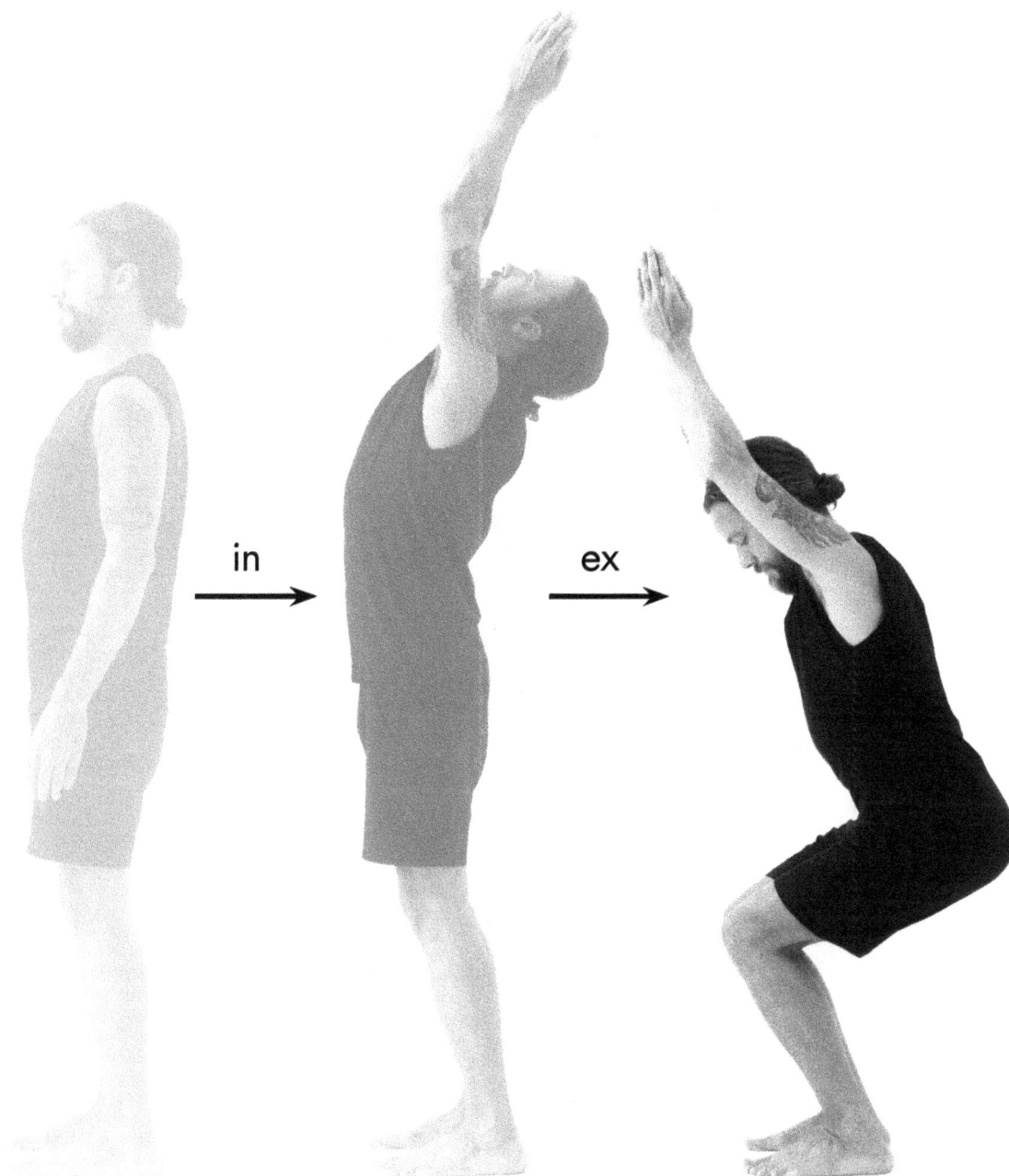

in → ex →

Move into other positions from the equal standing posture, following your breath each step of the way. Inhale for expanding, lengthening movements; exhale for contracting, bending movements.

arms overhead

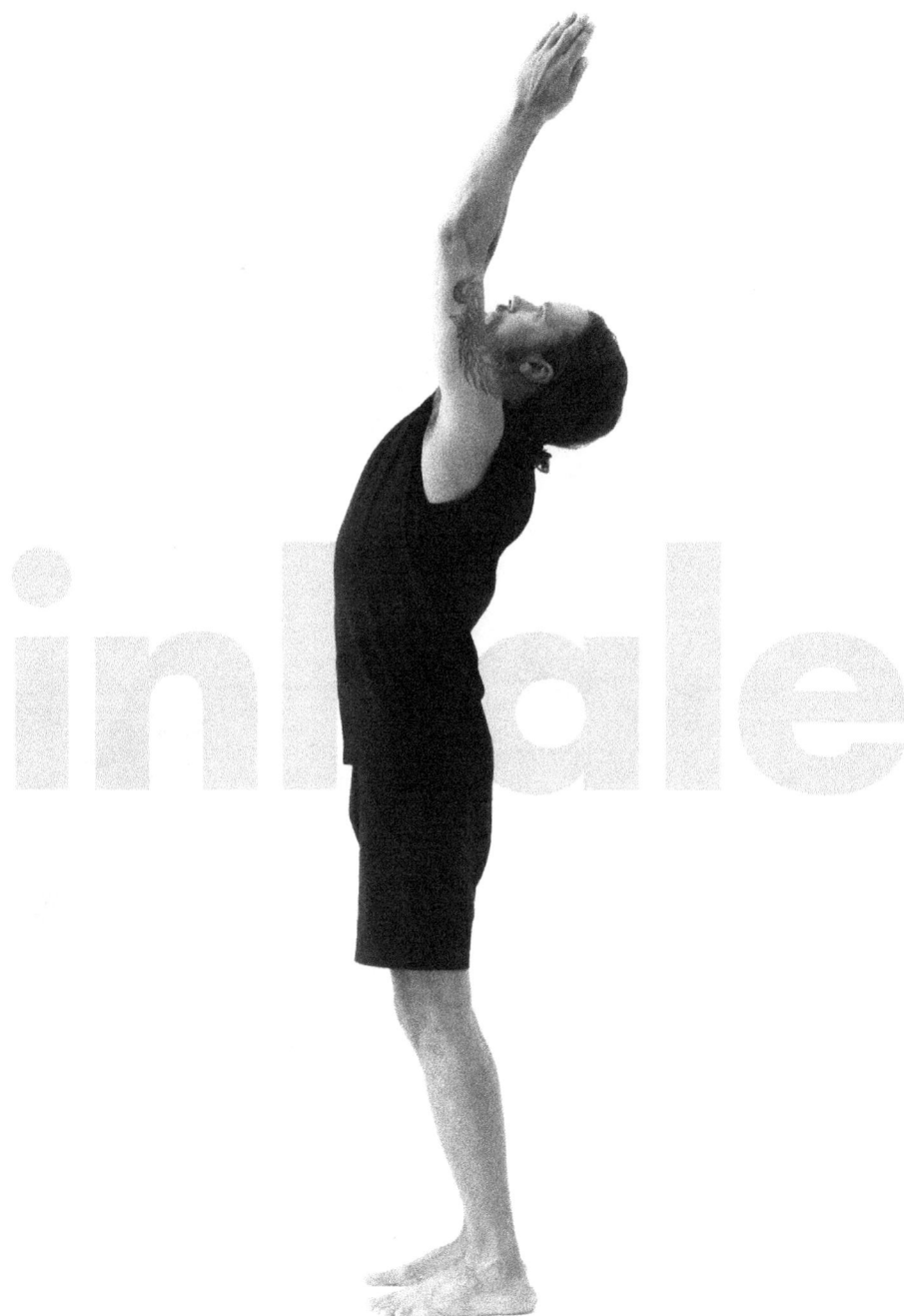

Inhale and sweep your arms out to the side and overhead, as though you're drawing a circle around your body with your chest at the center of the circle. Look up and see your hands come together. Allow your back to naturally arch as your chest fills with air.

exhale

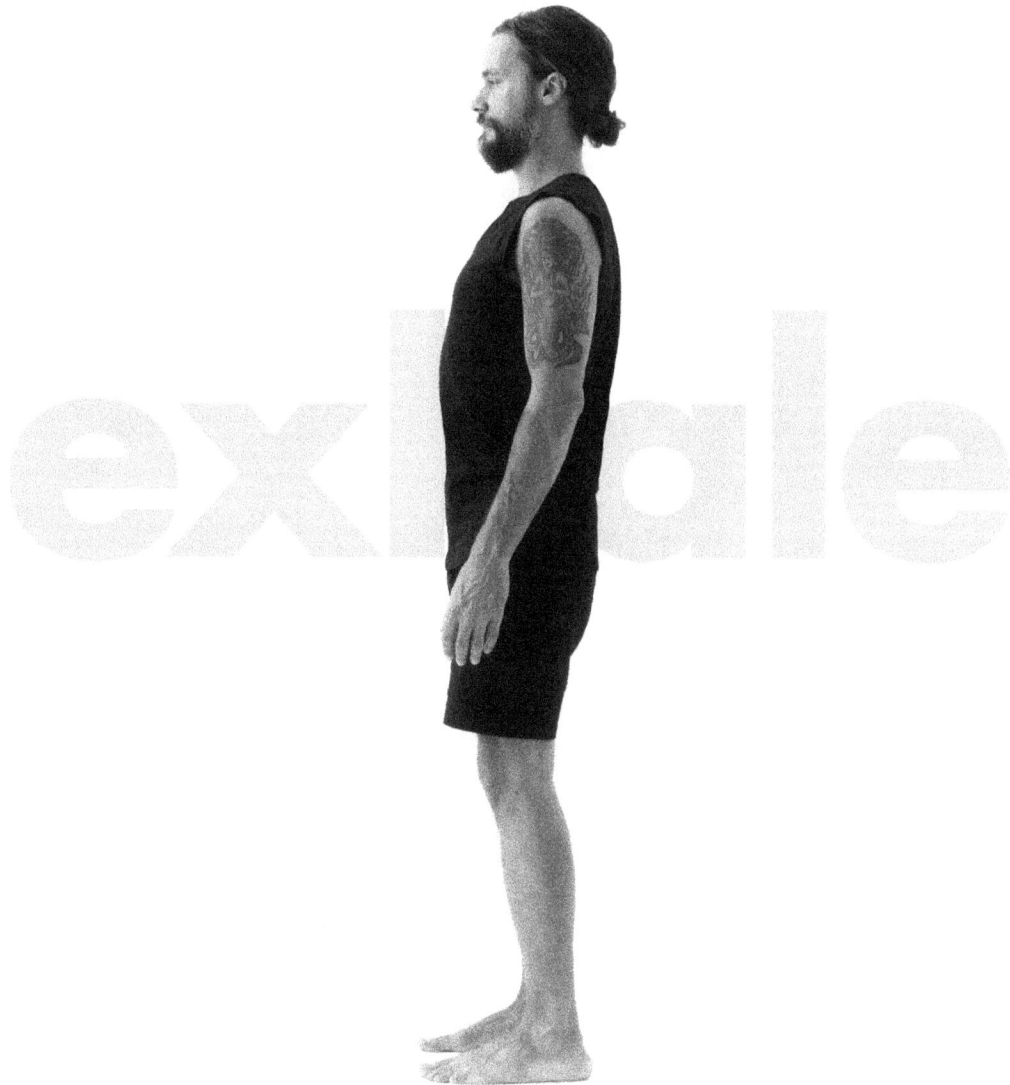

Exhale and gently contract your lower belly while returning your arms to your side, retracing the same circle you created on the inhalation. Allow your gaze to return to the horizon. Repeat the movement a number of times, focusing on keeping your breath slightly longer than the movement.

full body stretch

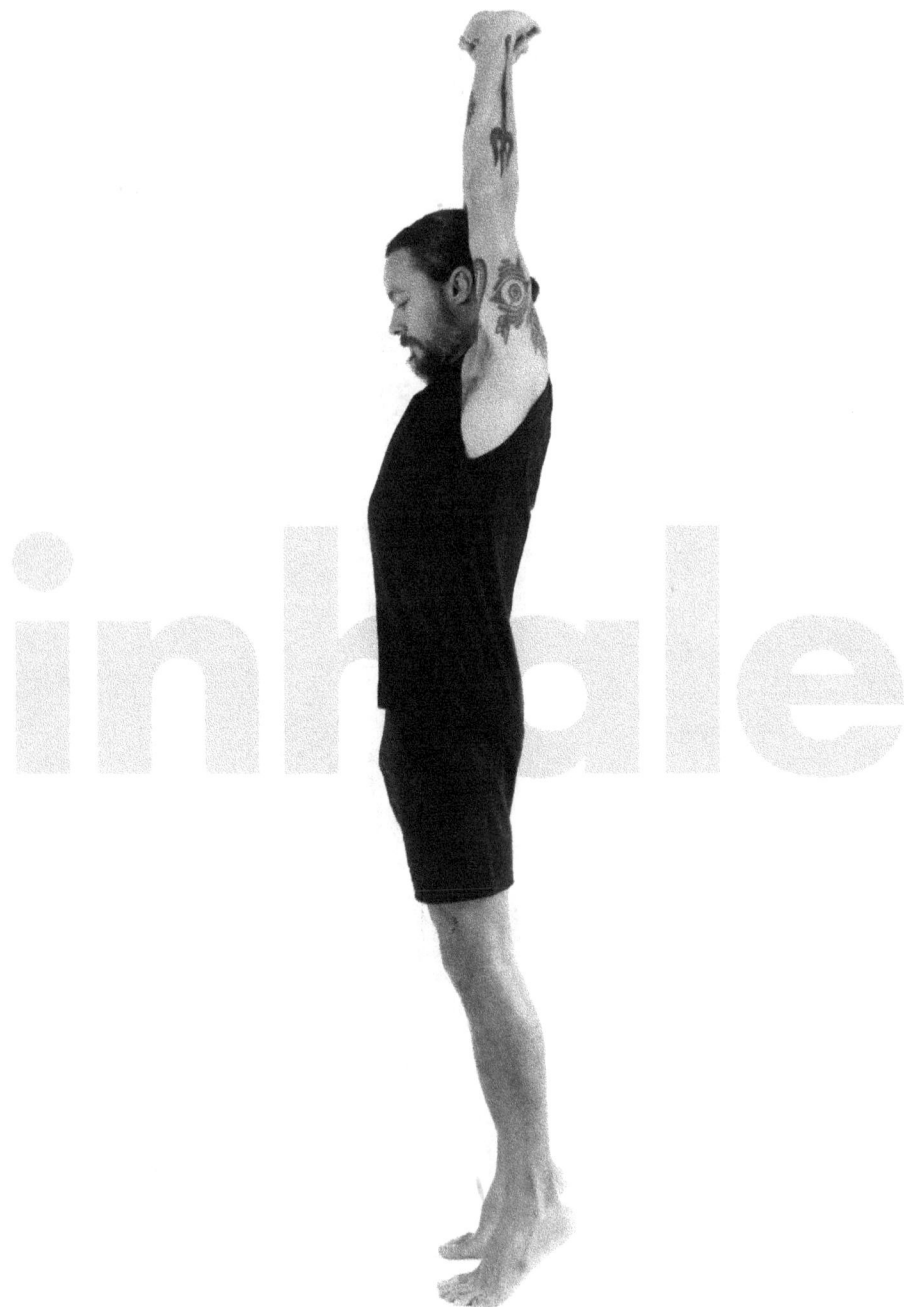

Inhale and sweep your arms out to the side and overhead, as though you're drawing a circle around your body with your chest at the center of the circle. At the top of the circle, interlace your fingers together with your palms turned up and stretch your arms. At the same time, lift your heels off the ground and balance on your toes.

exhale

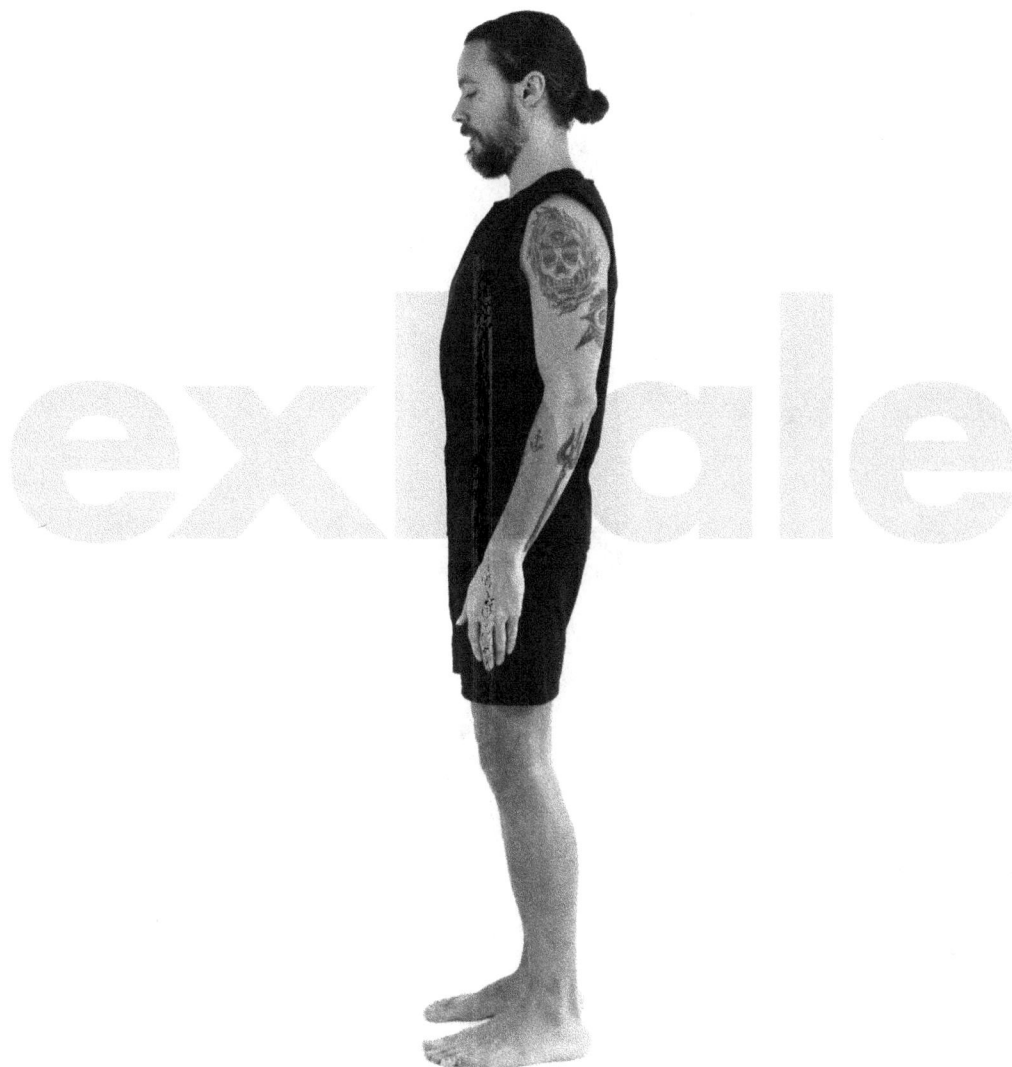

Exhale and gently contract your lower belly while returning your arms to your side, retracing the same circle you created on the inhalation. At the same time, lower your heels to the floor. Synchronize the movement of your arms with the raising and lowering of your heels. <u>Repeat</u> the movement a number of times. <u>Stay</u> in the lifted 'inhale' position for a number of breaths.

standing twist

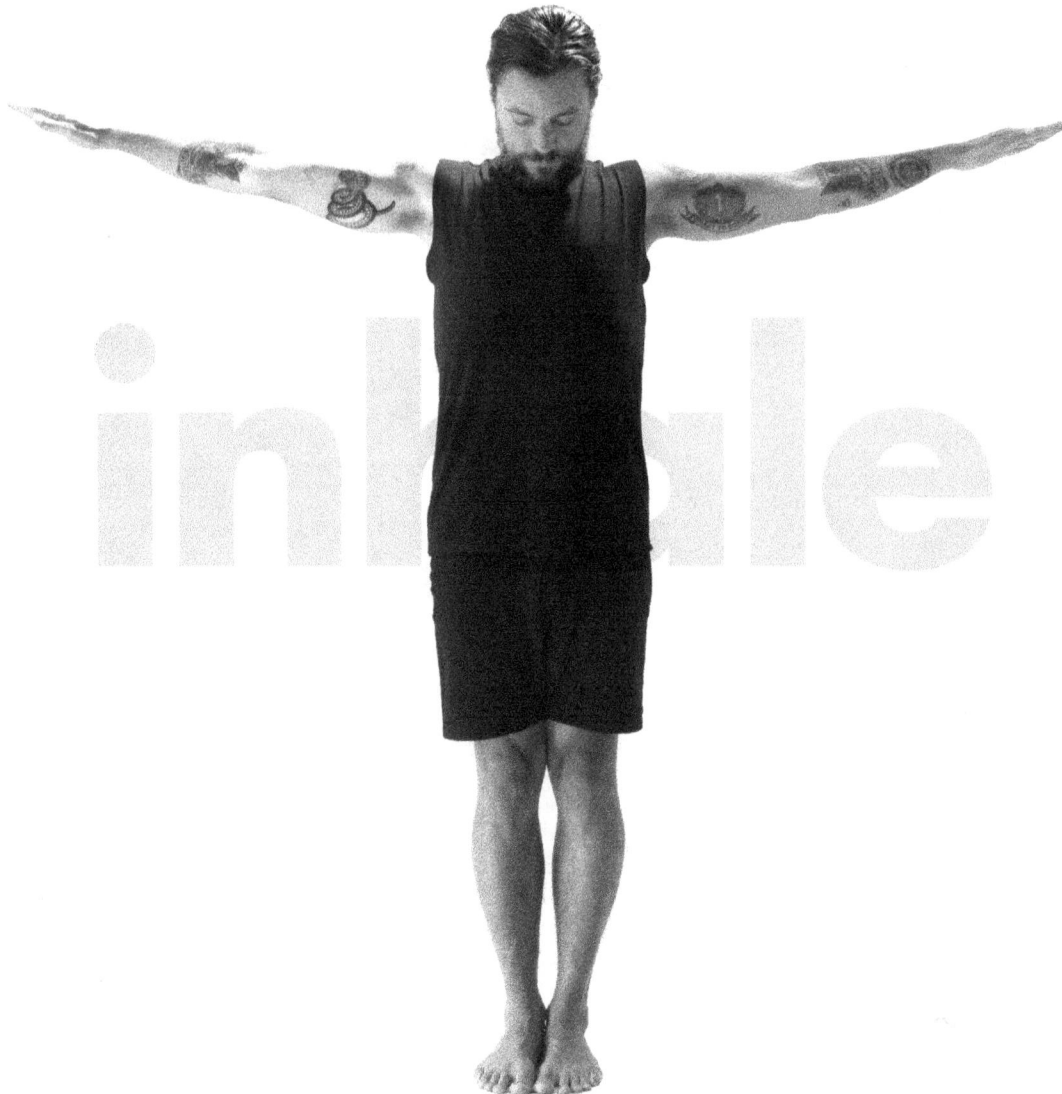

Inhale and raise your arms shoulder height and parallel to the ground. Keep your chin lowered to meet your rising chest. <u>Try this</u>: Perform the movement with your feet at varying distances from each other to feel the difference.

exhale

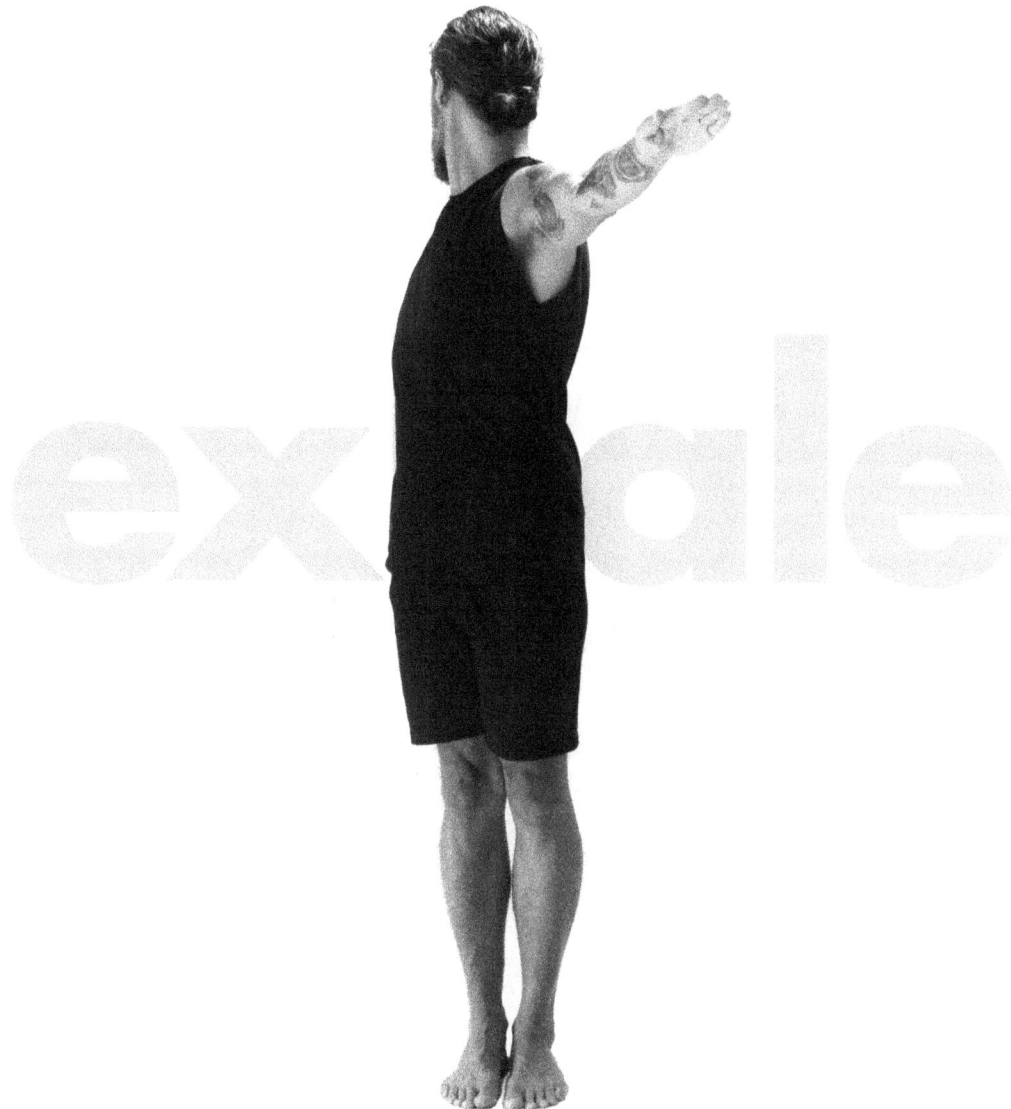

Exhale, turn and look over your shoulder, keeping your feet firmly planted on the ground. Keep your arms parallel to the ground and your chest open. Pause for a moment in the twist before inhaling and returning to the starting position. Repeat the movement a number of times, alternating sides with every exhale. Stay in the 'exhale' position for an equal number of breaths on each side.

forward bend

inhale

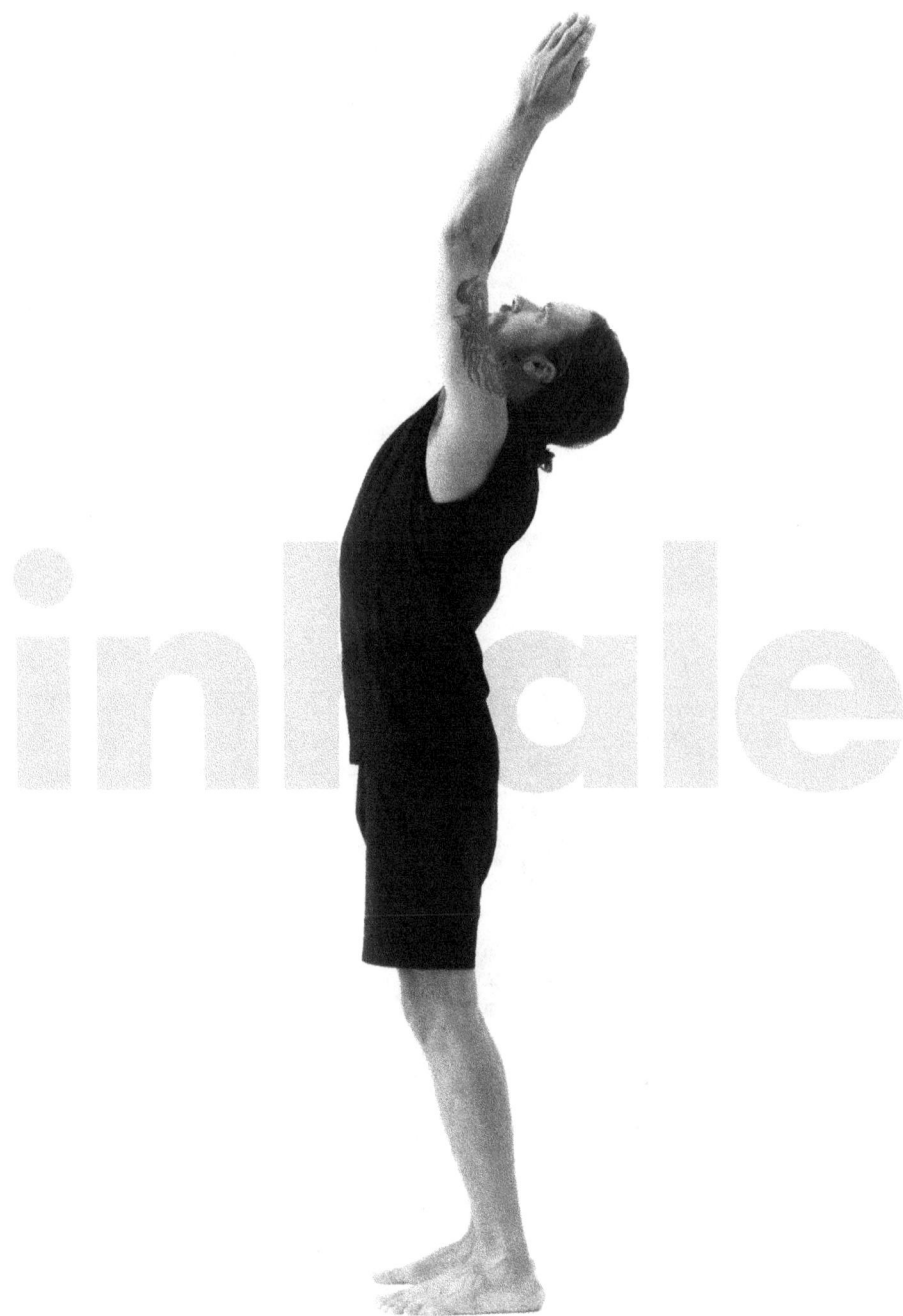

Inhale as you sweep your arms in a circle around your body, chest lifting into a gentle back arch. Look up and see your hands come together overhead. Engage your backside muscles to help support the back arch.

exhale

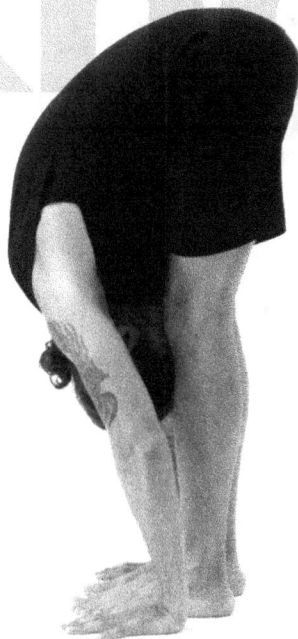

Exhale and draw in your lower abdominals as you hinge forward at your waist. Follow your exhalation all the way down. Bend your knees enough so that you can comfortably touch the ground. Repeat the movement a number of times. Stay in the 'exhale' position for a number of breaths; every inhalation allow your spine to lengthen and chest expand; every exhalation draw in your abdominals and release more deeply into the forward bend.

halfway lift

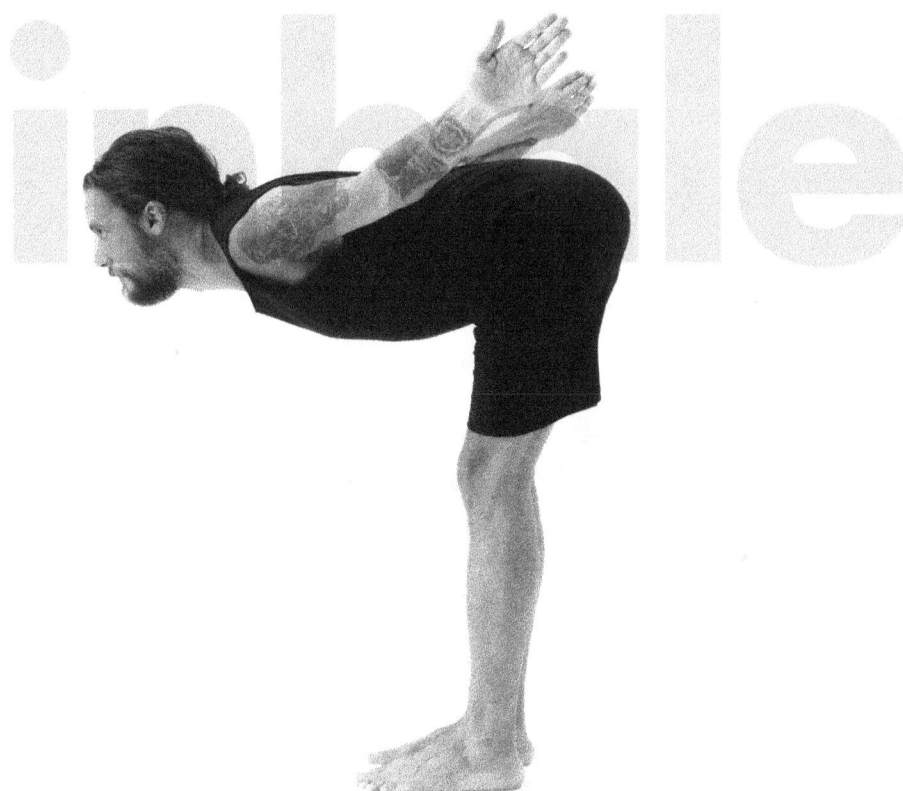

Getting there: Start in the forward bend position from the previous spread.
Inhale and lift your chest and torso parallel to the ground, arms sweeping back and legs straightening. Extend from the crown of your head to your tailbone, and lift your upper chest. <u>Modify</u> if necessary by using your hands on your shins for support. <u>Try</u> reaching your arms forward as you lift up to make the movement more challenging.

exhale

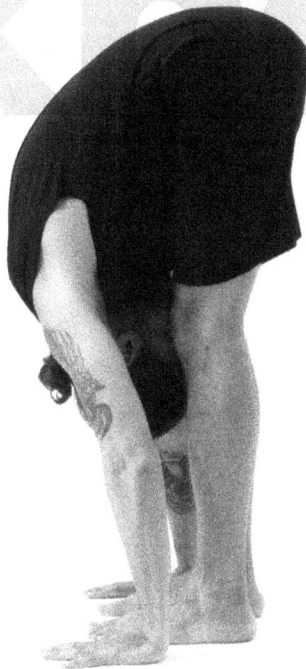

Exhale and hinge forward at your waist, bending your knees as much as needed to avoid straining. <u>Repeat</u> the movement a number of times. <u>Stay</u> in the 'inhale' position for a number of breaths, only if you are comfortable. It may take some time to develop the strength to do this safely.

half squat

inhale

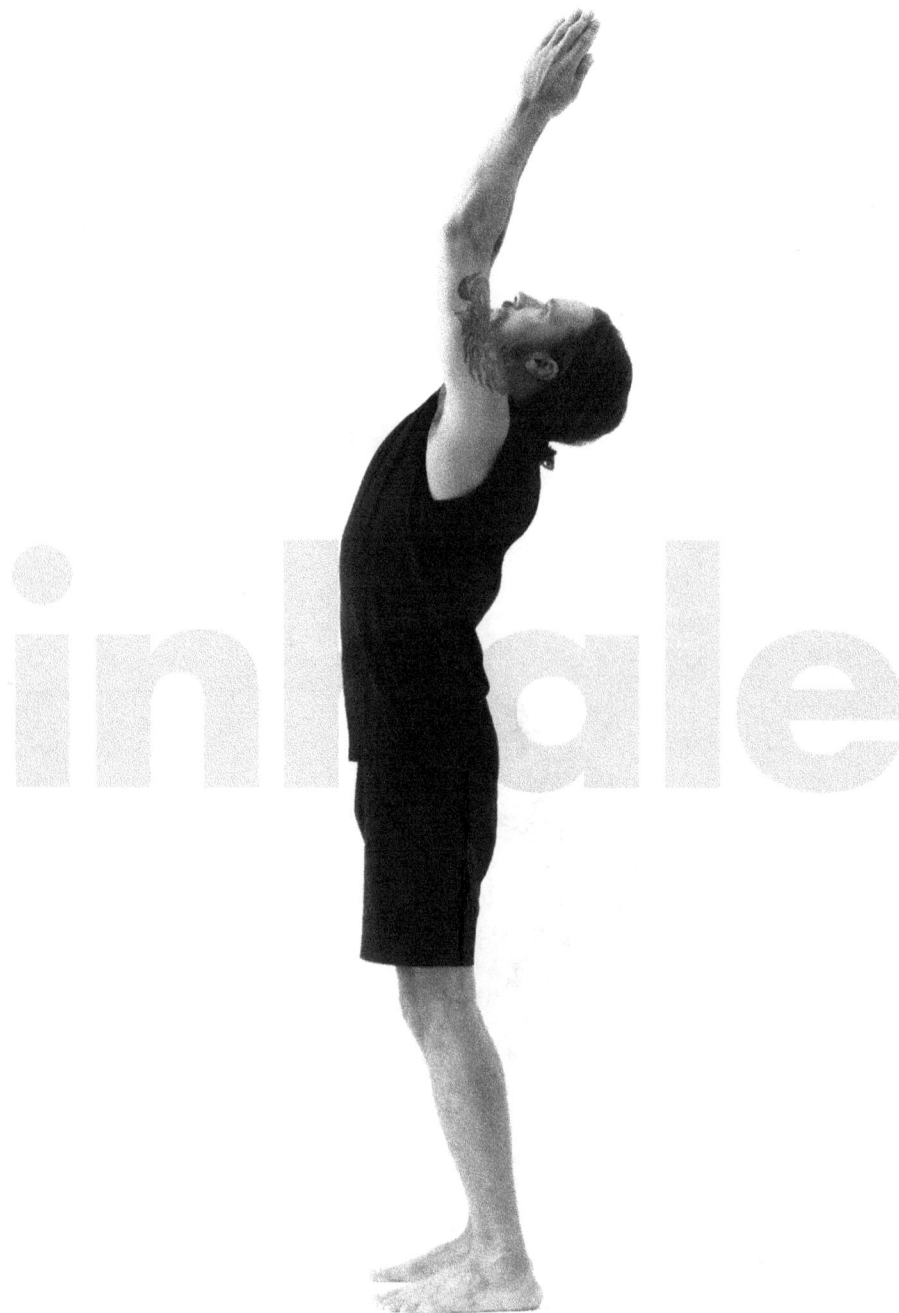

Inhale and sweep your arms in a circle around your body, opening up into a gentle back arch. See your hands come together overhead.

exhale

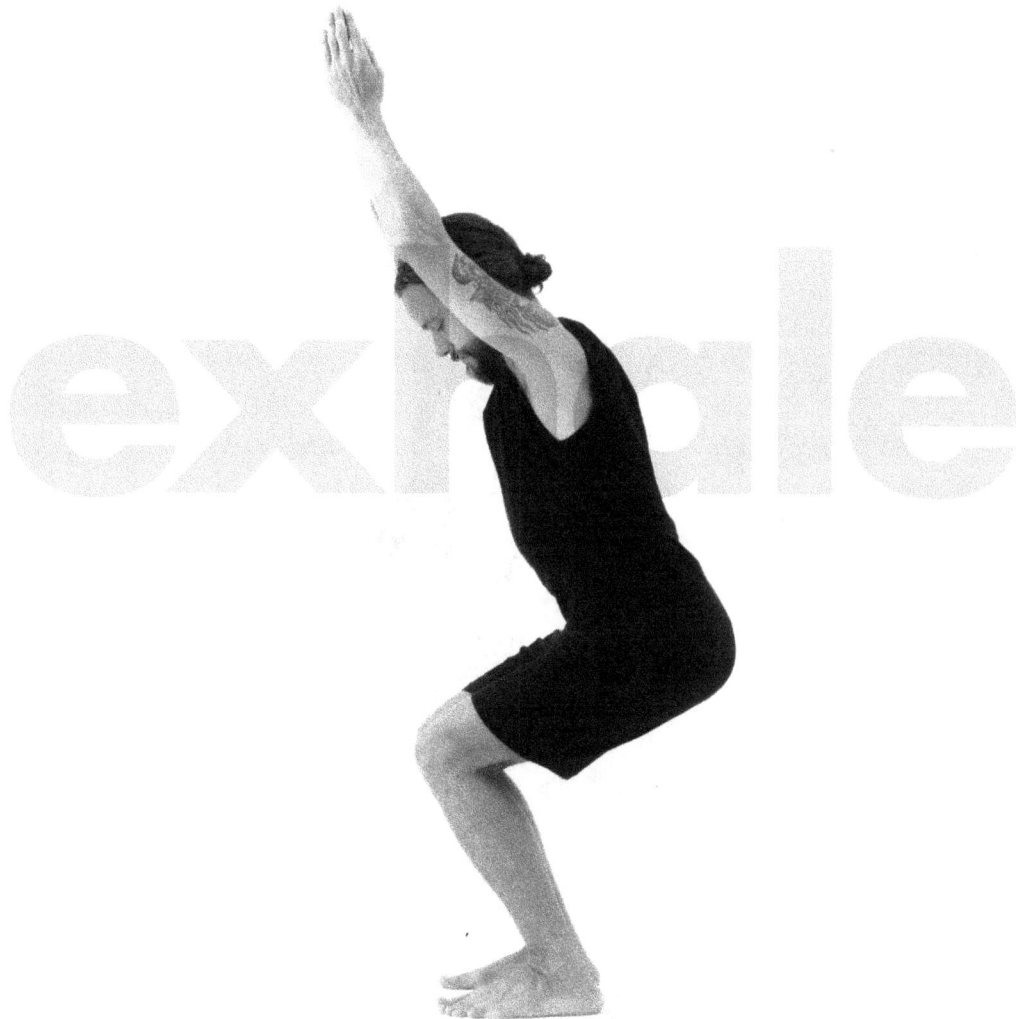

Exhale and sit down into a half squat, arms overhead. Keep your knees steady.
You should still be able to see your toes in front of your knees. Pause and focus on keeping your
knees steady and feet firmly connected to the ground. Repeat the movement a number of times.
Stay in the 'exhale' position for a number of breaths (see next spread for instruction).

half squat stay

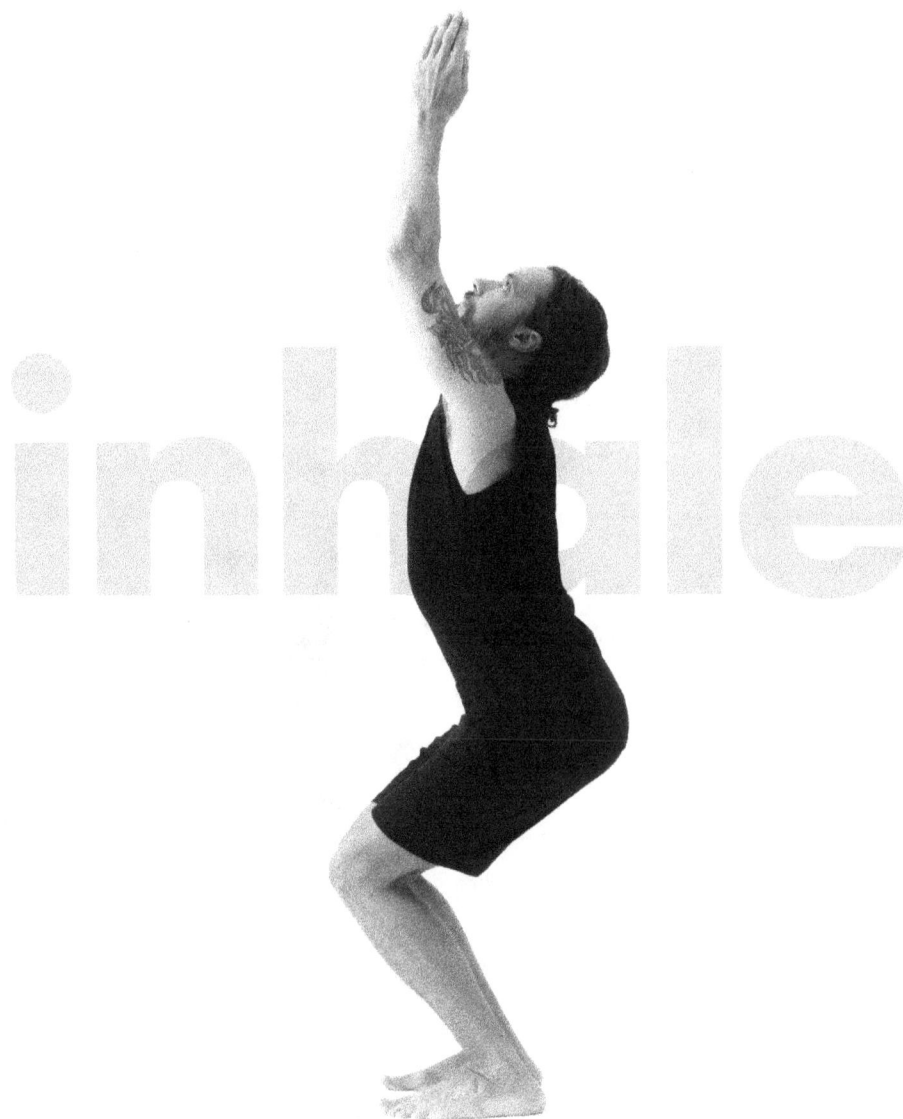

Getting there: From the equal standing position, inhale and bring your arms overhead. Exhale and sit down in a half squat (this is the exhale position).
Inhale and lift your chest, looking up. If you're not comfortable lifting your head in this position, keep looking forward.

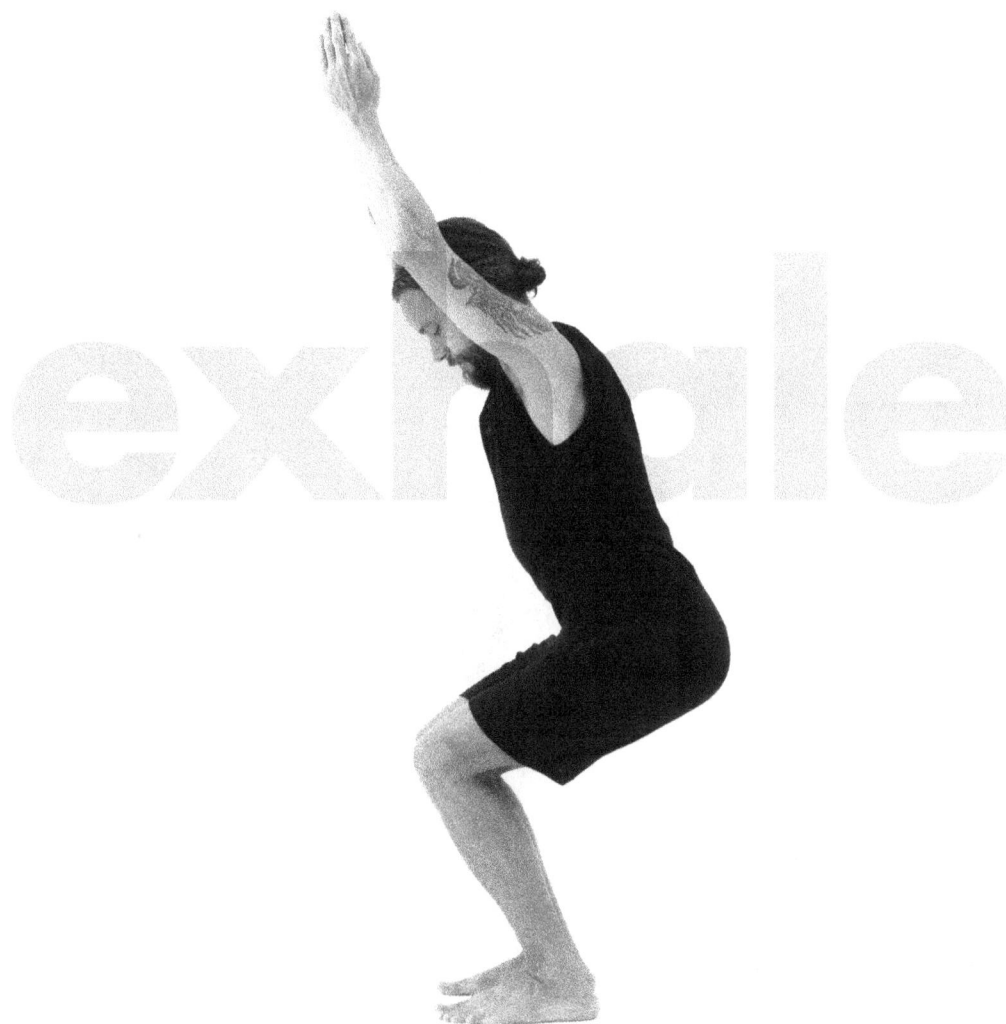

Exhale and let your upper back and chest relax a little, bringing your gaze downward.
As you continue to inhale and exhale in the half squat, feel your breath as a wave-like movement
in your spine. Repeat the movement a number of times, then return to standing on inhalation.

deep squat

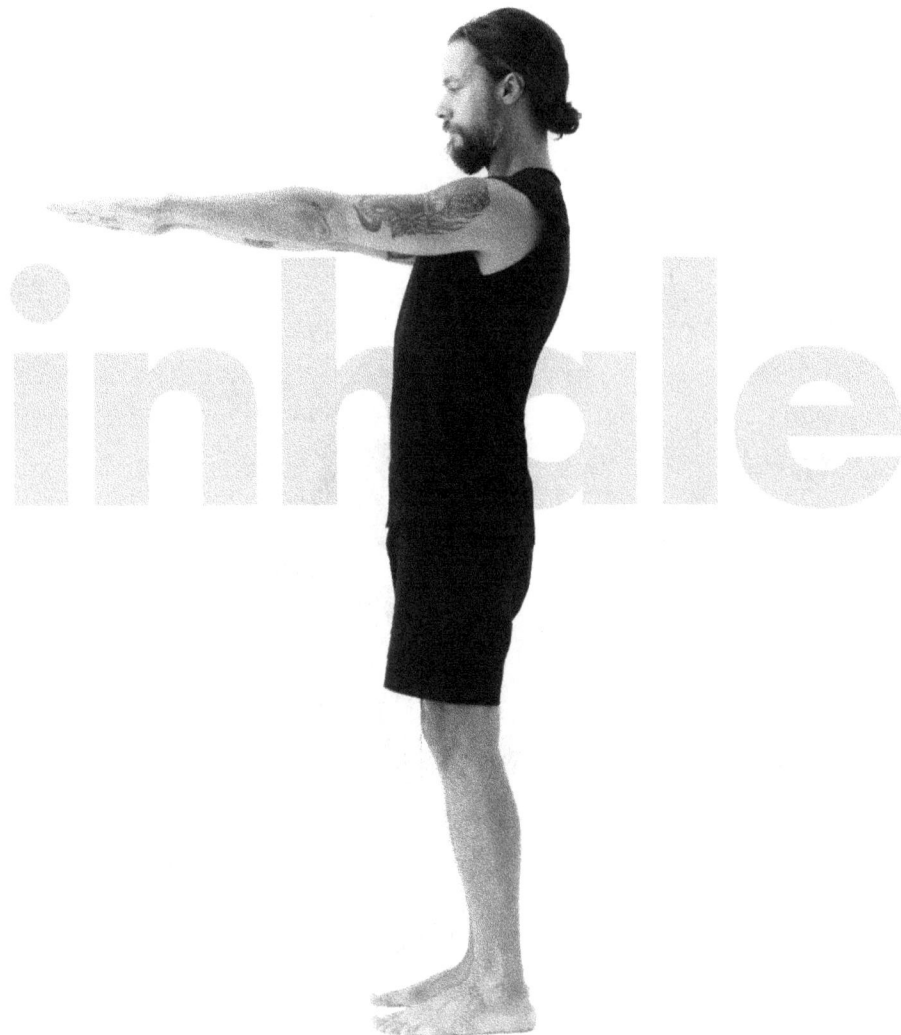

Inhale and bring your arms up in front of you, shoulder height and parallel to the ground, palms facing down. <u>Modify</u> if necessary by widening your stance, or raising your heels. You can also perform this movement holding on to a railing for support until you develop more strength and mobility.

exhale

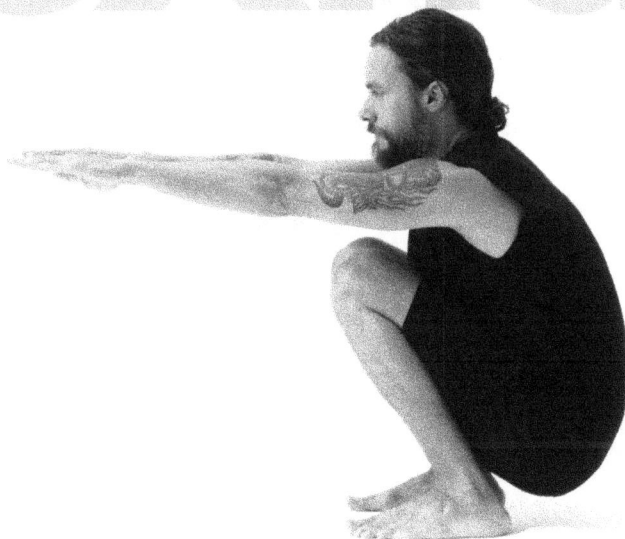

Exhale and sit down as low as you can comfortably, keeping your arms in front for balance. Avoid letting your knees go past your toes. <u>Repeat</u> the movement a number of times. <u>Stay</u> in the 'exhale' position for a number of breaths.

striding forward bend

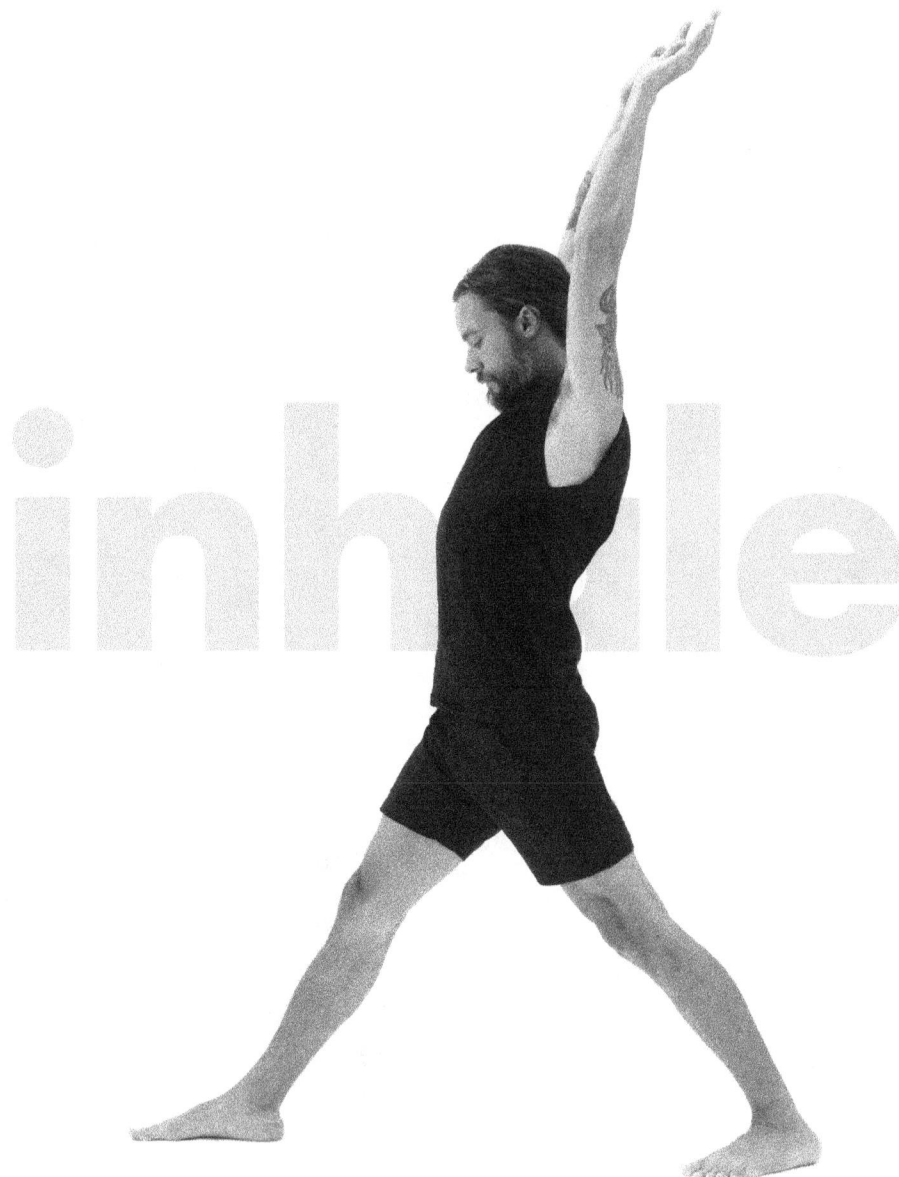

Getting there: From the equal standing position, stride one leg back about 3-4 feet, keeping your feet hip width. Allow your back foot to turn out about 45°.
Inhale and lift your arms up in front of your body. Keep your chin lowered toward your chest.

exhale

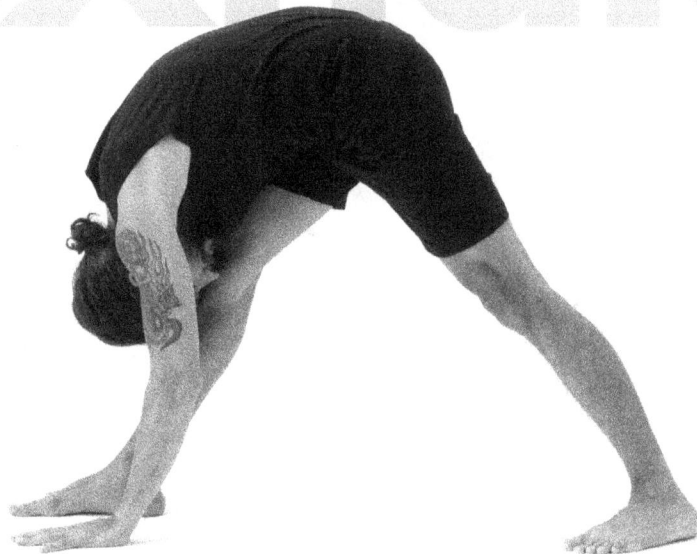

Exhale and hinge at the waist, keeping your arms outstretched and spine extended until your head is close to your knee. Avoid locking out your joints, and bend your forward knee as much as you need to avoid strain. <u>Repeat</u> the movement a number of times. <u>Stay</u> in the 'exhale' position for a number of breaths, then repeat the sequence on the other side.

warrior

inhale

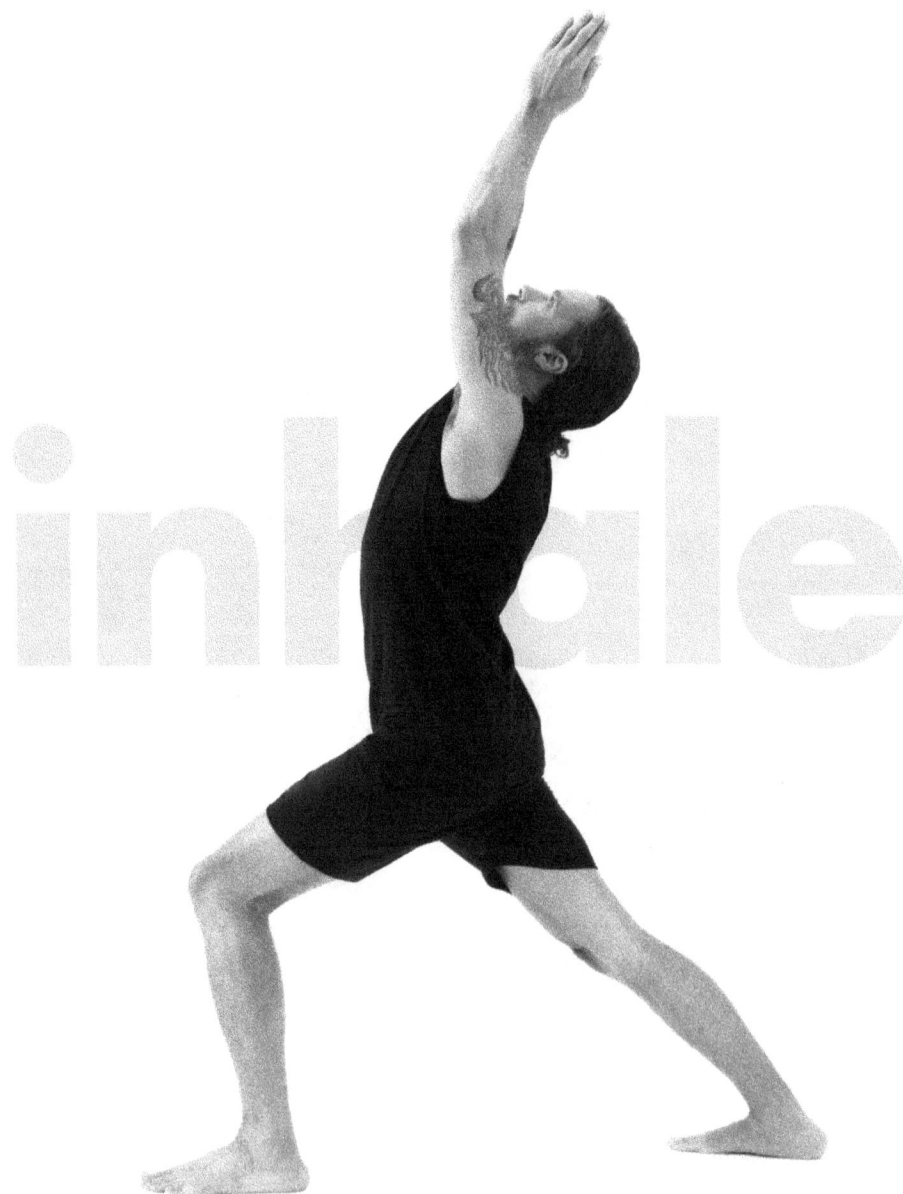

Getting there: From the equal standing position, stride one leg back about 3-4 feet, keeping your feet hip width. Allow your back foot to turn out to avoid strain in your hips. Bend your front knee 45°- 90°.

Inhale and sweep your arms up in a circle around your body, lifting your gaze to see your hands come together overhead.

exhale

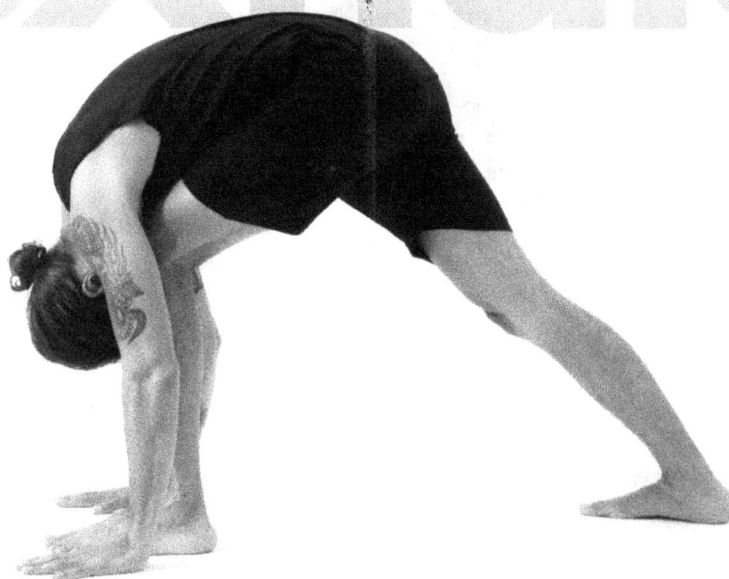

Exhale and draw in your lower abdominals as you hinge forward, bringing your hands to the ground, retracing the circular motion of your arms. Relax your head as you pause. <u>Repeat</u> the movement a number of times. <u>Stay</u> in the 'inhale' position for a number of breaths, then repeat the sequence on the other side.

forward bend & twist

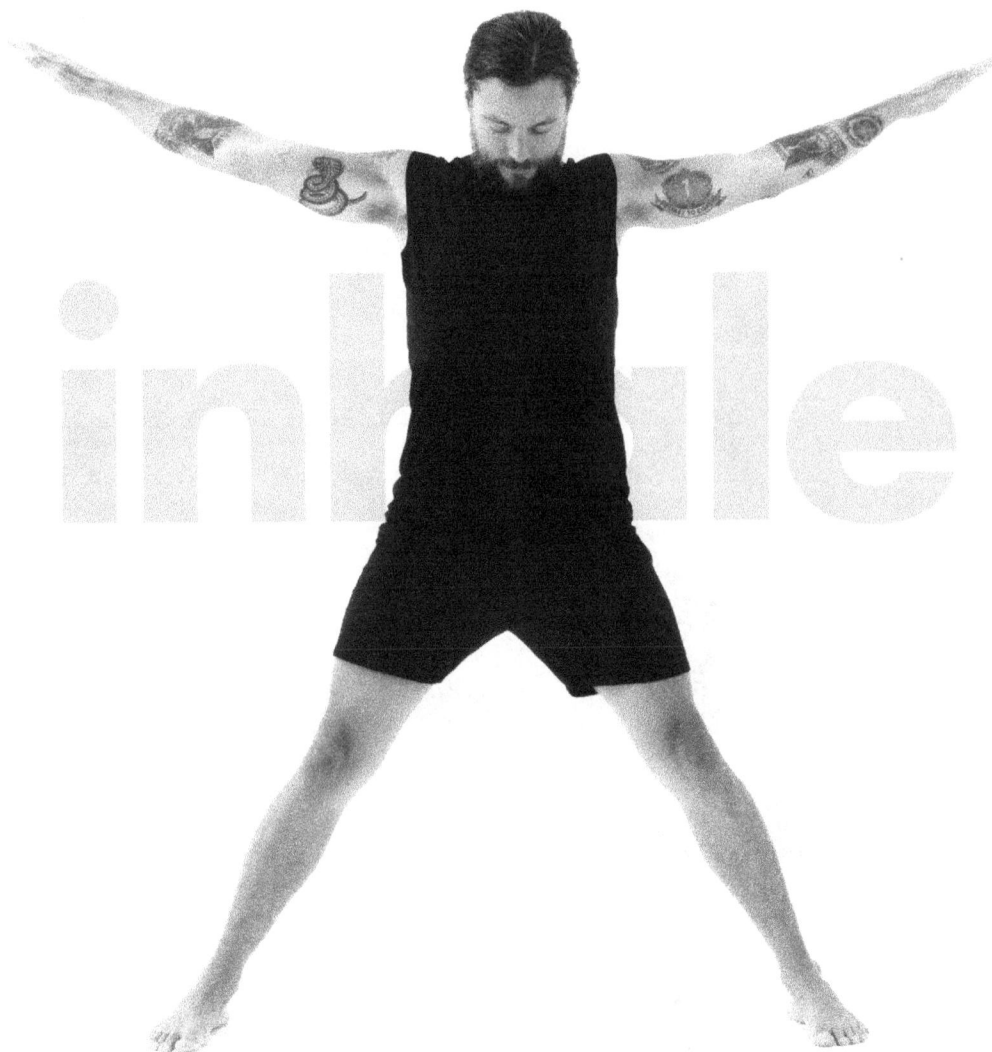

Getting there: From the equal standing position, step or jump your feet apart wider than your shoulders but still steady and stable.

Inhale and raise your arms parallel to the ground, keeping your chin down.

exhale

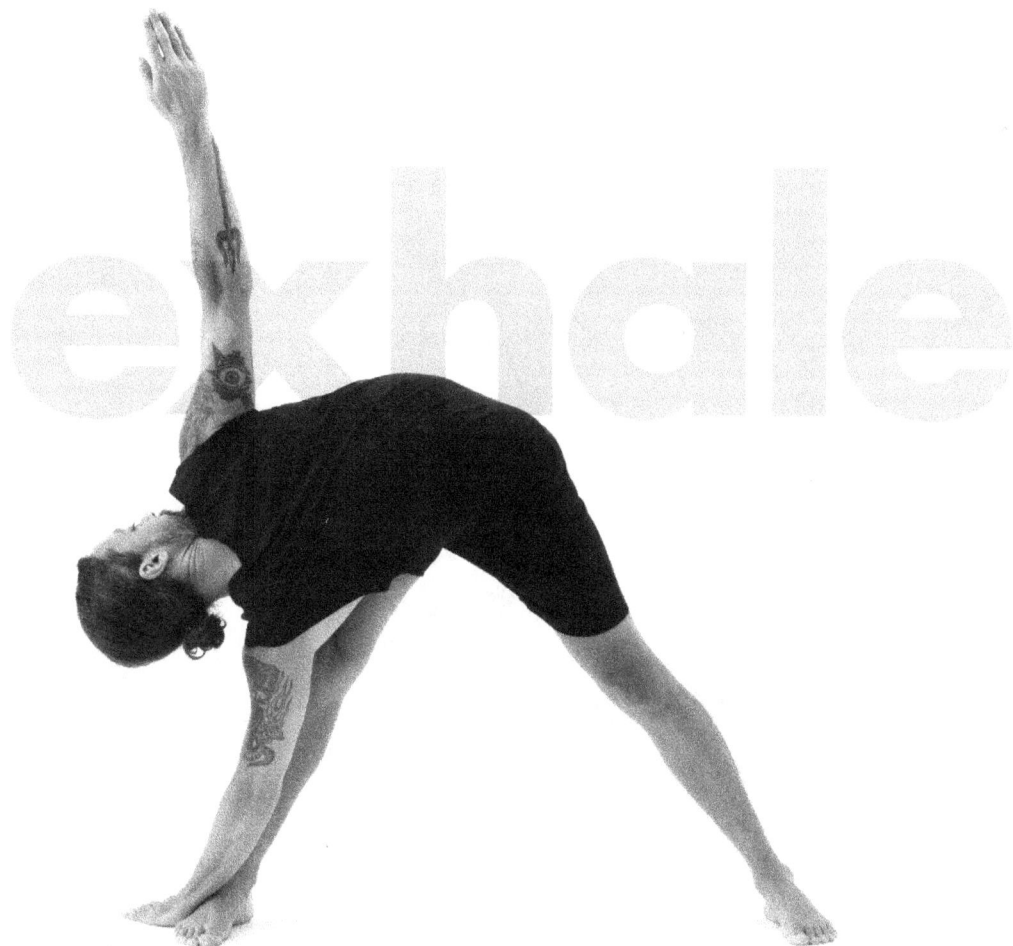

Exhale and bend forward, simultaneously twisting and bringing your hand to the opposite foot or shin. Turn your head and look up to your top hand. <u>Repeat</u> the movement a number of times, alternating sides. Inhale up, exhale twist. <u>Stay</u> in the 'exhale' position for an equal amount of time on each side. <u>Modify</u> if necessary by bending the knee that you're twisting toward. If shoulder mobility is an issue you can try bringing your upper hand to your lower back.

squat twist

inhale

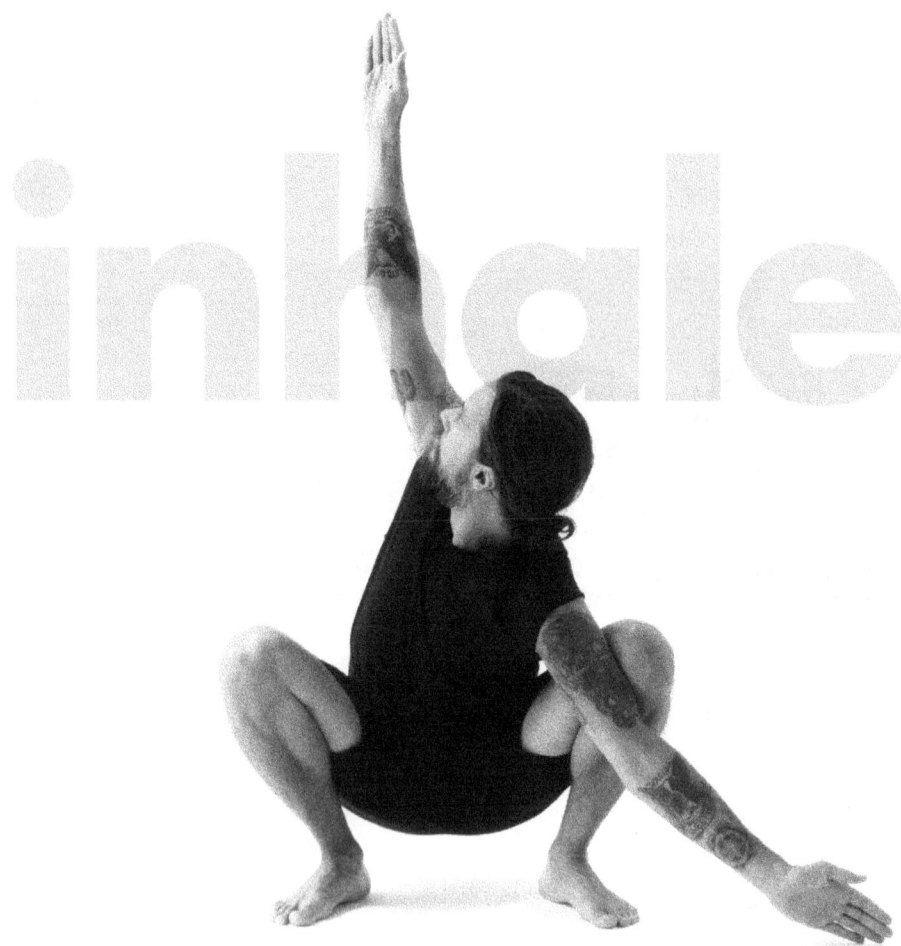

Getting there: Begin standing with feet a little wider than shoulder distance, hands together in front of your chest. Exhale as you lower into a full squat, turning your feet out as needed. **Inhale** as you twist to one side and open your arms — one to the ground, the other to the sky. Turn your head to look at your top hand. <u>Modify</u> if necessary by placing a small rolled towel under your heels.

exhale

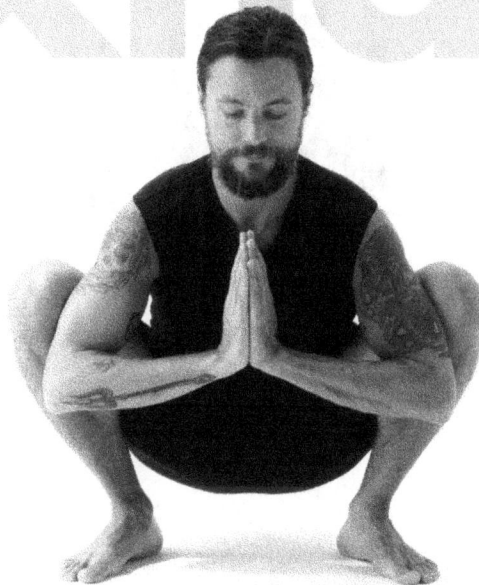

Exhale and return to the starting position bringing your hands together in front of your chest.
<u>Repeat</u> the movement a number of times, alternating sides. Inhale twist, exhale return to center.
<u>Stay</u> in the 'inhale' position for an equal amount of time on each side.

side angle stretch

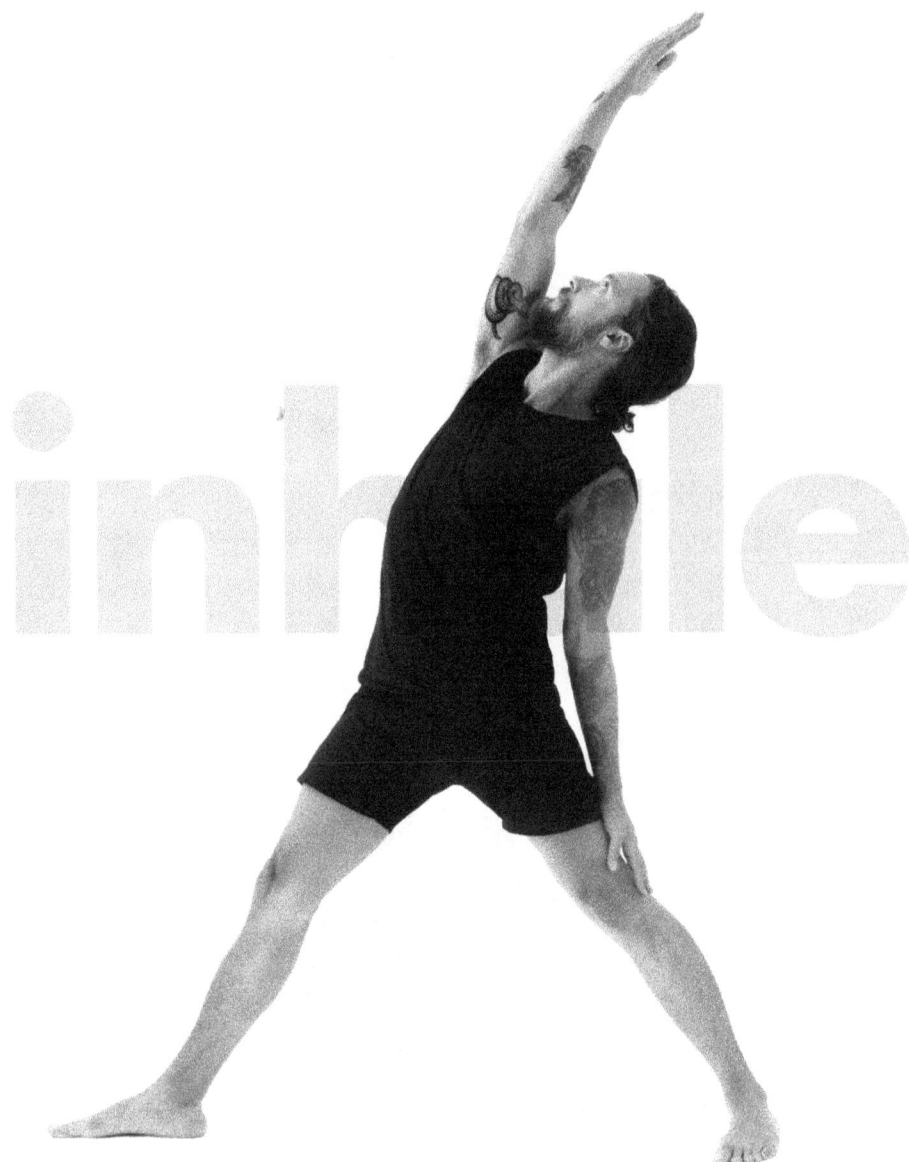

Getting there: Start in a wide stance and turn one foot out 90°.
Inhale and raise the arm on the same side as your out-turned foot and stretch it up overhead.
Your other hand can rest on your rear leg for support.

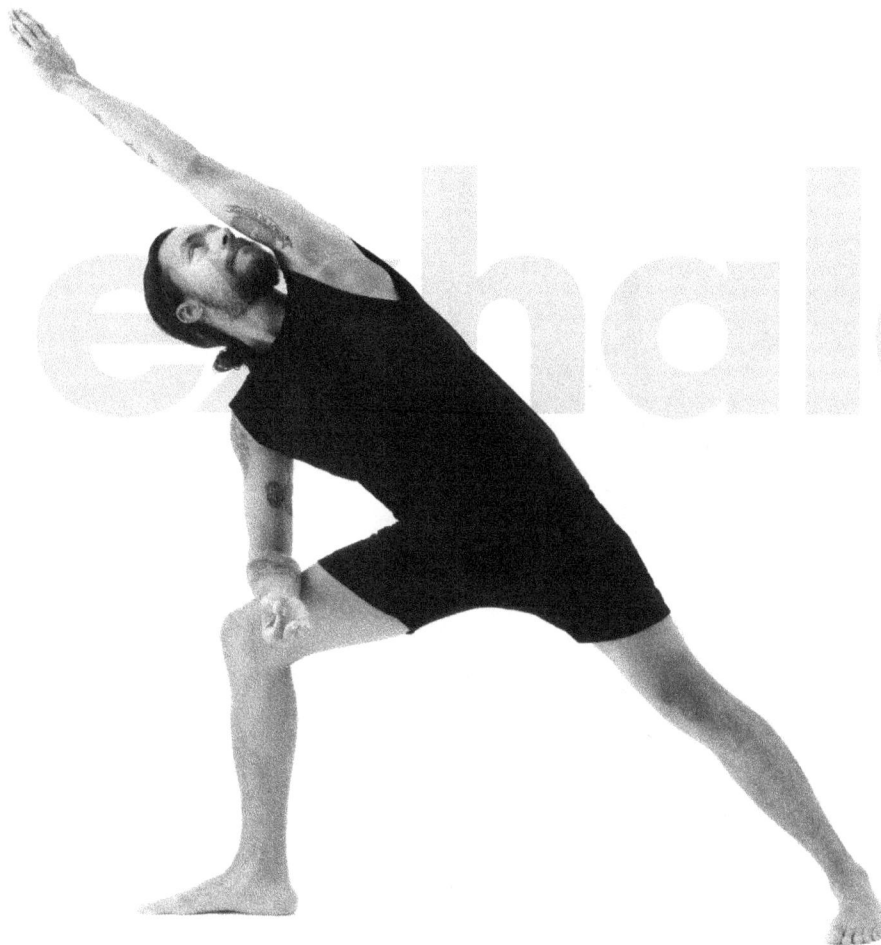

Exhale as you lower the arm that was lifted and bend your leg on that side so that your forearm can rest on your thigh. Alternately, you can bring that hand to the floor. Sweep the opposite arm up overhead and feel a stretch through that side. <u>Repeat</u> the movement a number of times. <u>Stay</u> in the 'exhale' position for a number of breaths, then repeat the sequence on the other side.

one leg balance

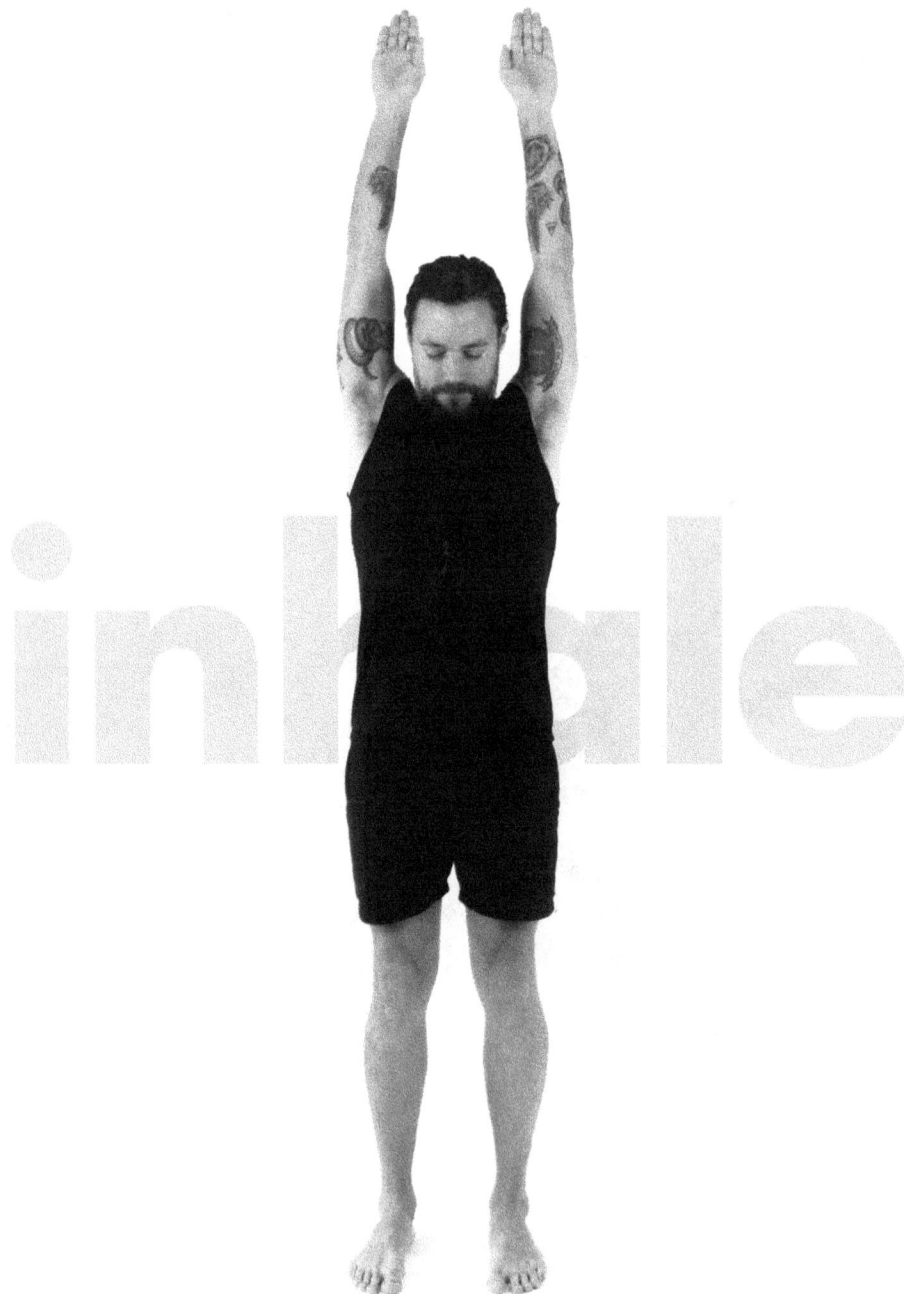

inhale

Getting there: Start in the equal standing position, feet hip width and parallel, arms resting at your sides.

Inhale as you raise your arms straight up overhead, keeping your chin down.

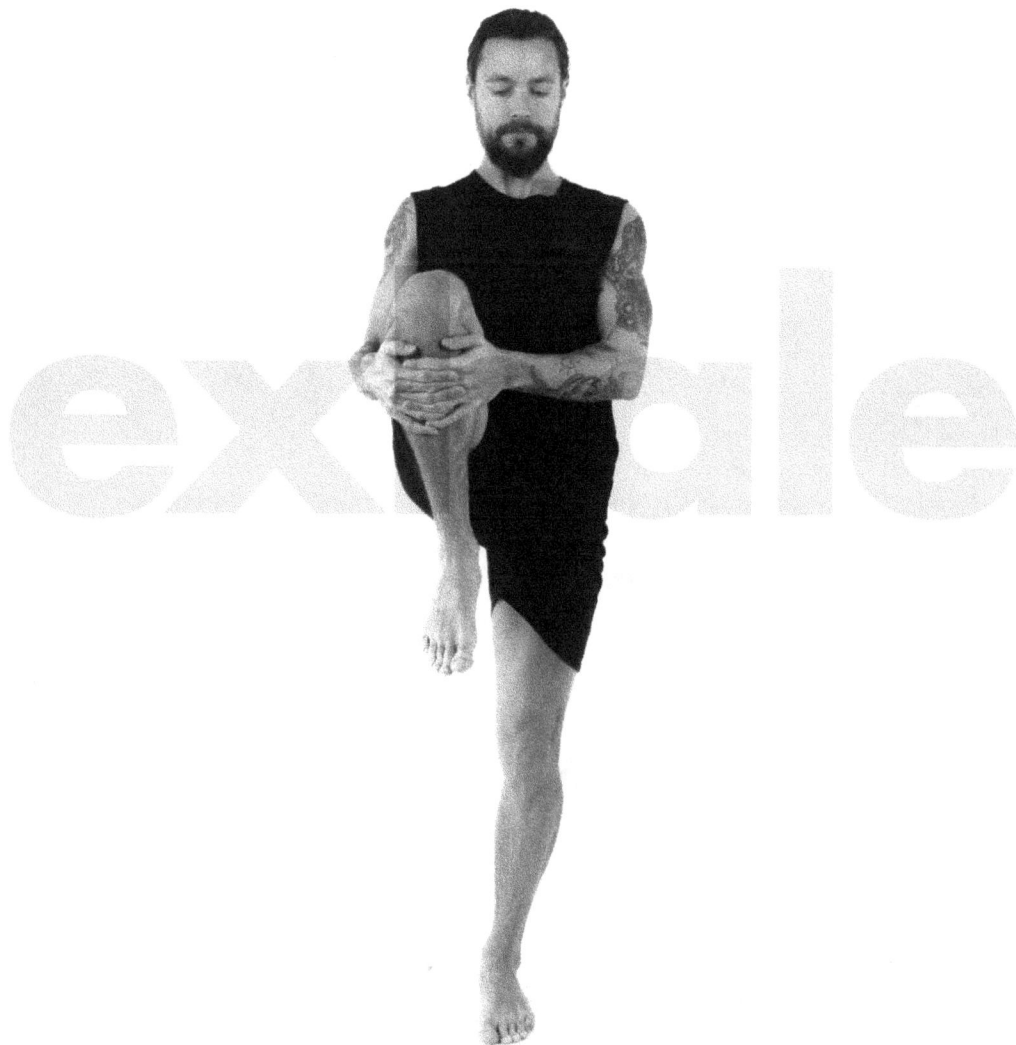

Exhale as you lift one knee toward your chest, taking your hands to your shin and giving a gentle squeeze in. <u>Repeat</u> the movement a number of times, alternating legs. Inhale stretch up, exhale draw your knee in. <u>Stay</u> in the 'exhale' position for an equal number of breaths on each side.

3.2 transition movements

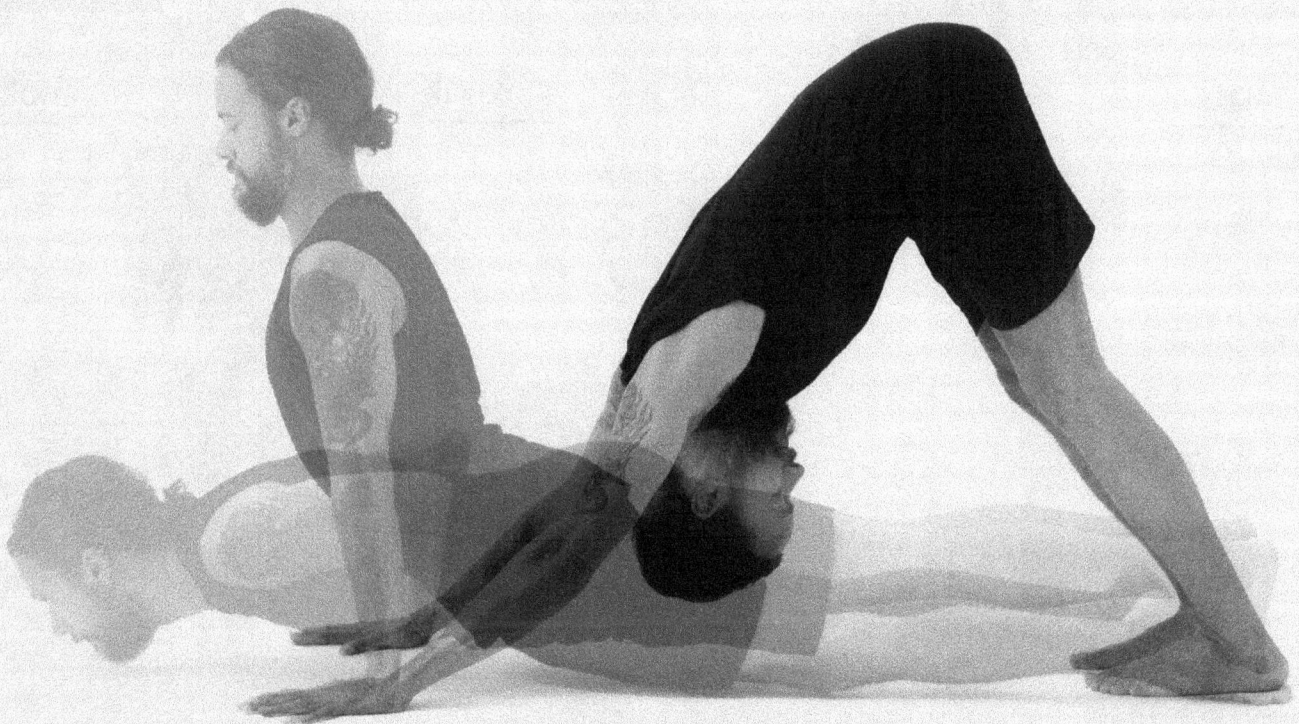

standing to kneeling

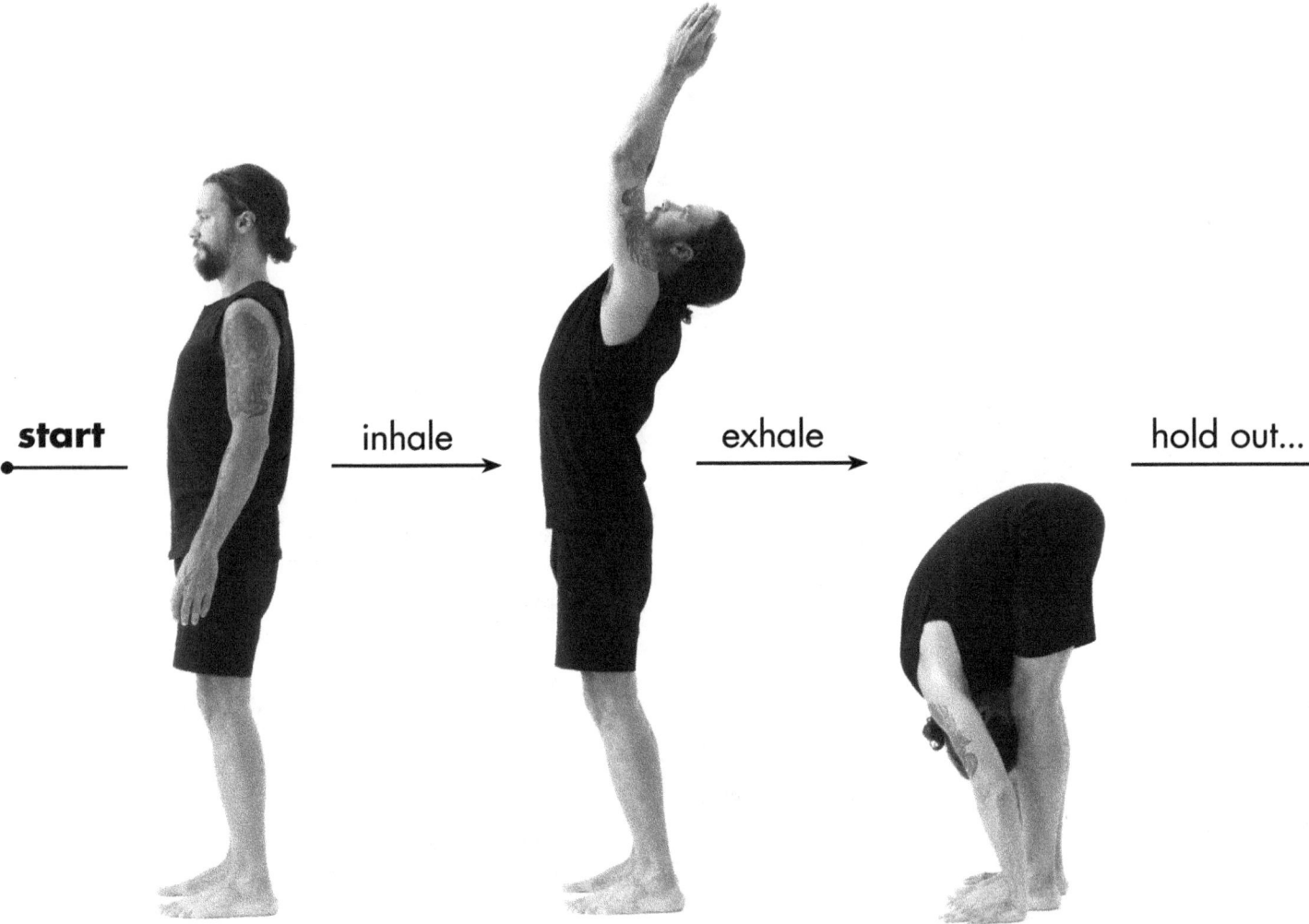

start → inhale → exhale → hold out...

...step back → inhale → **finish** →•

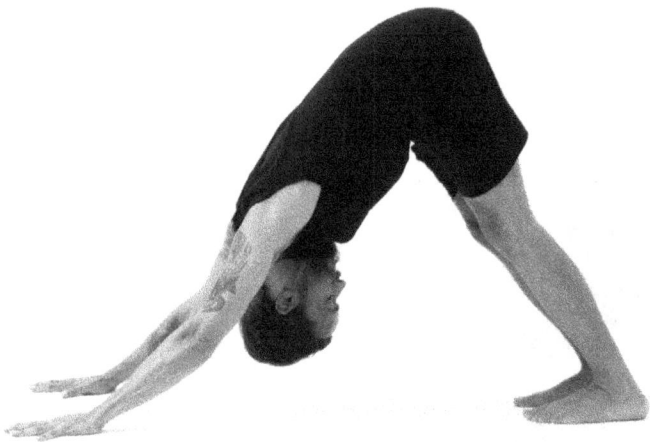 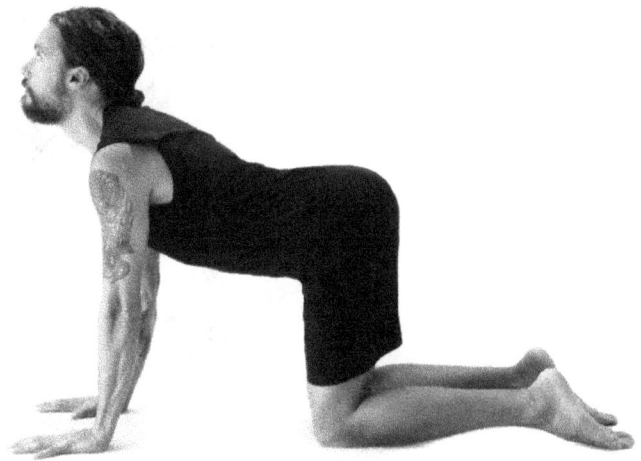

back arch to down dog

inhale

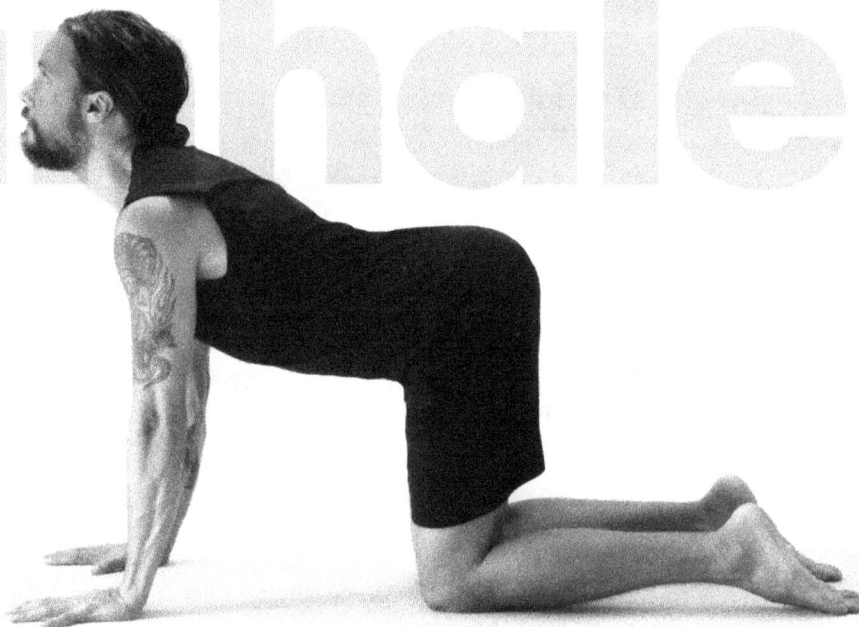

Getting there: From the equal standing posture, inhale and raise your arms overhead. Exhale into a forward bend bringing your hands to the floor, shoulder distance. Step or hop both feet back about 4 feet. Inhale and lower your knees to the floor (see previous spread). **Inhale** and expand your chest as you lift your head and arch your back.

exhale

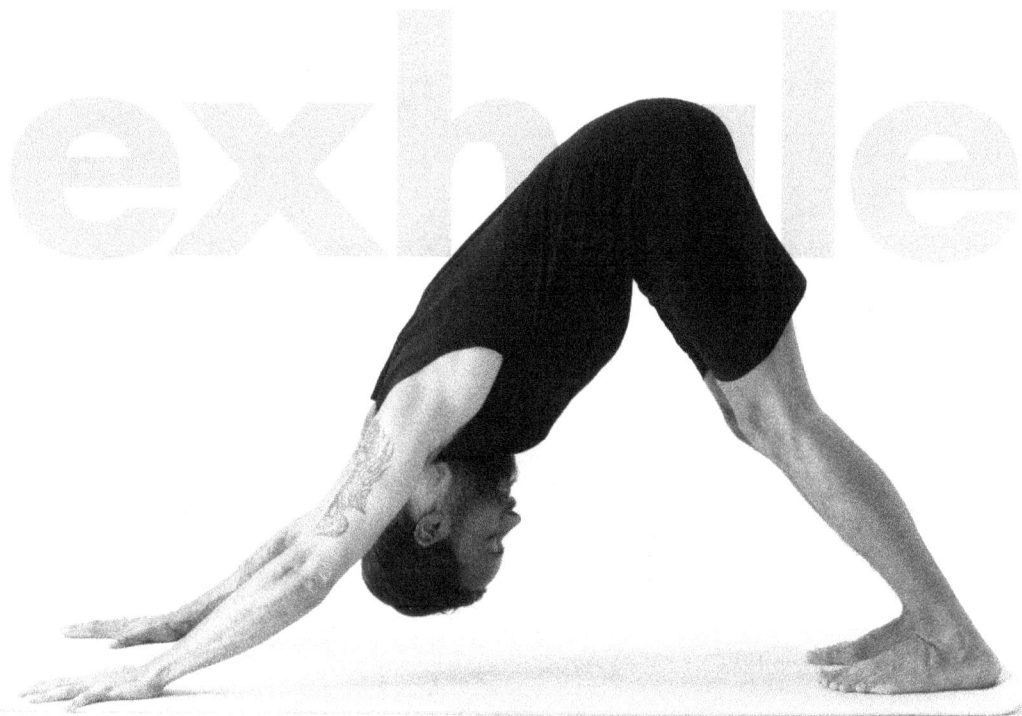

Exhale as you push your hips up and back, straightening your arms and lengthening your spine. At first, it may help to keep your knees bent and heels off the floor. Repeat the movement a number of times. Stay in the 'exhale' position for a number of breaths.

up dog to down dog

inhale

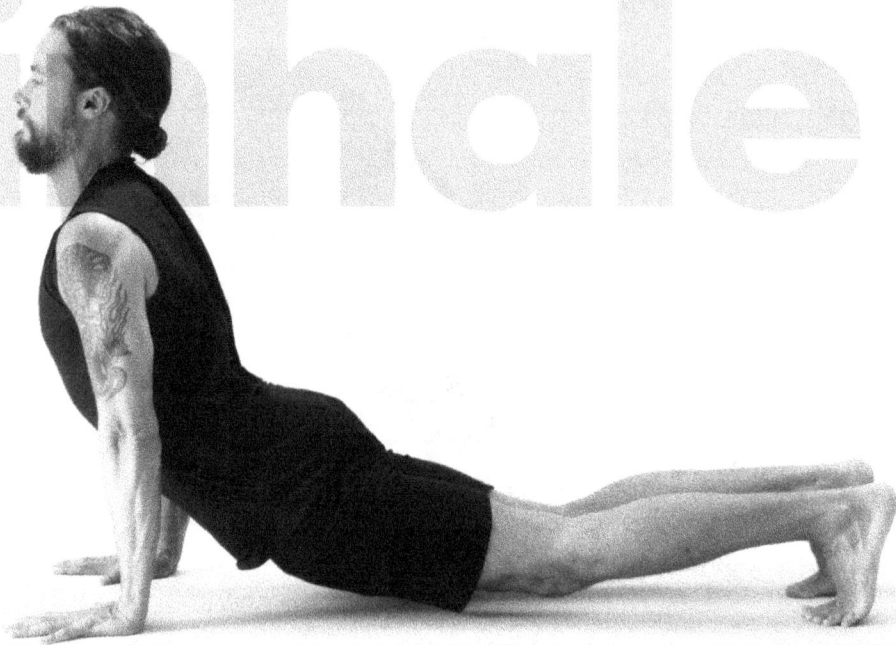

Getting there: Following the previous instructions, find your way into down dog. **Inhale** and bring your chest forward until your arms are perpendicular to the ground. Keep your toes tucked under and thighs off the floor.

exhale

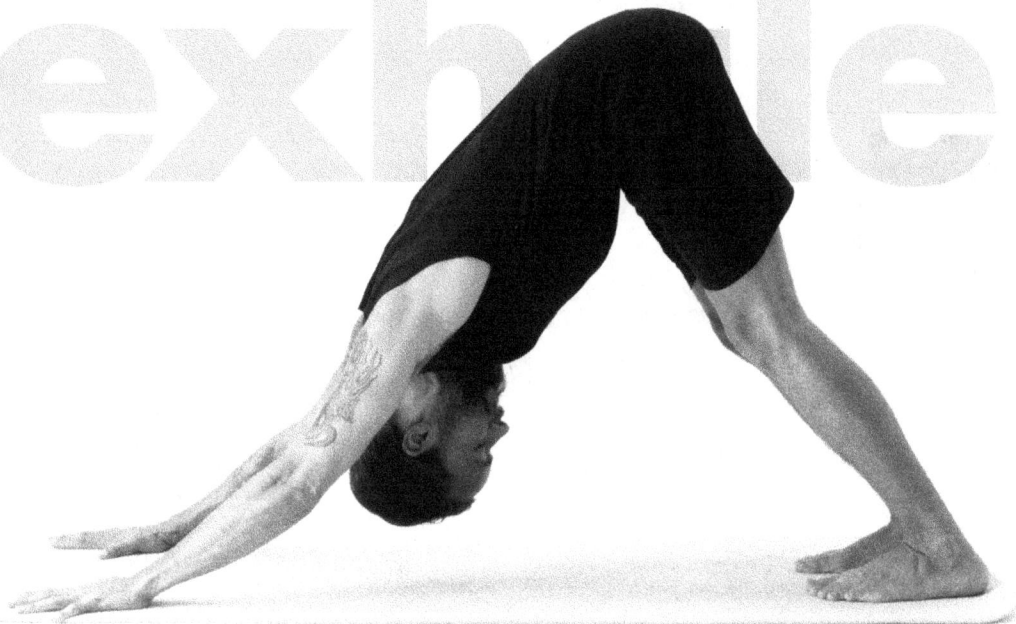

Exhale and push your hips up and back, returning to the down dog position. Repeat the movement a number of times. Inhale up dog, exhale down dog. Stay in both the 'inhale' and 'exhale' position for an equal number of breaths.

plank pushup

inhale

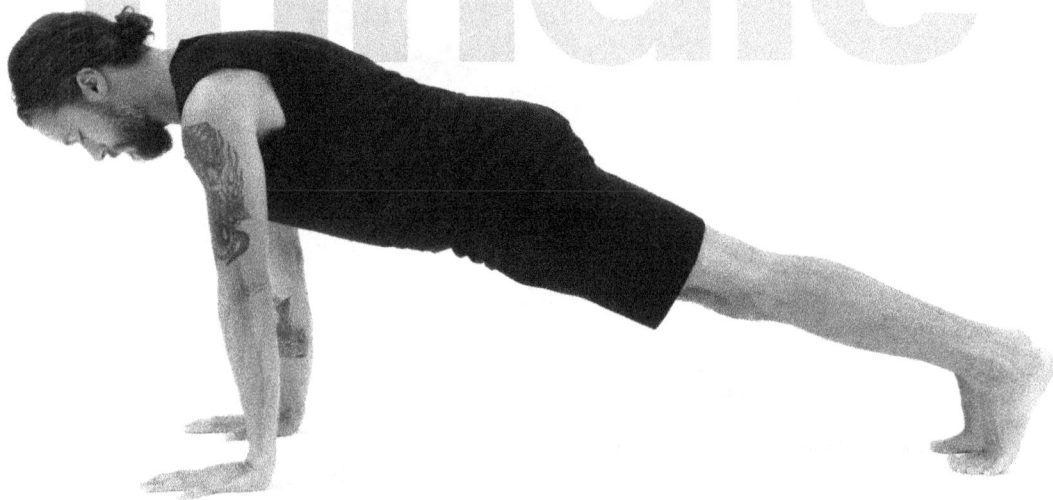

Getting there: From the forward bend position, hold your breath out as you hop or step back into a plank position, with shoulders over your wrists, back and legs in a straight line.
Inhale and straighten your arms, keeping your belly firm and hands engaged. Modify if necessary by keeping your knees on the ground for support.

exhale

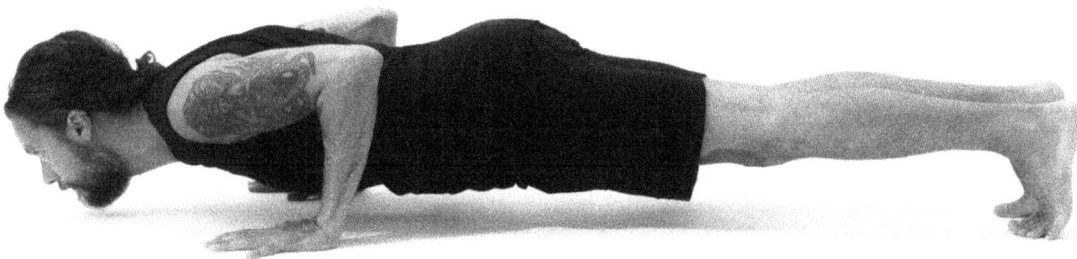

Exhale and lower down until your legs and torso are in a straight line parallel to the ground. Keep your elbows close to your sides. <u>Repeat</u> the movement a number of times. <u>Stay</u> in each position for a number of breaths.

3.3 kneeling movements

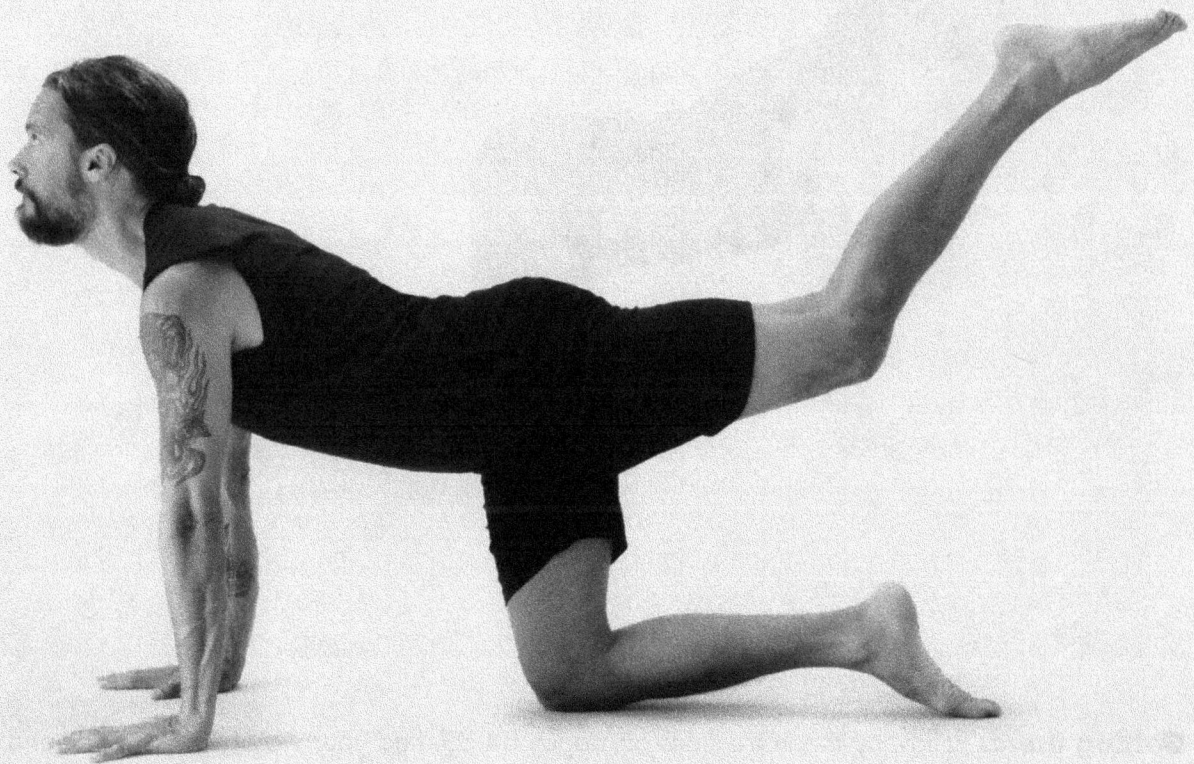

spinal waves

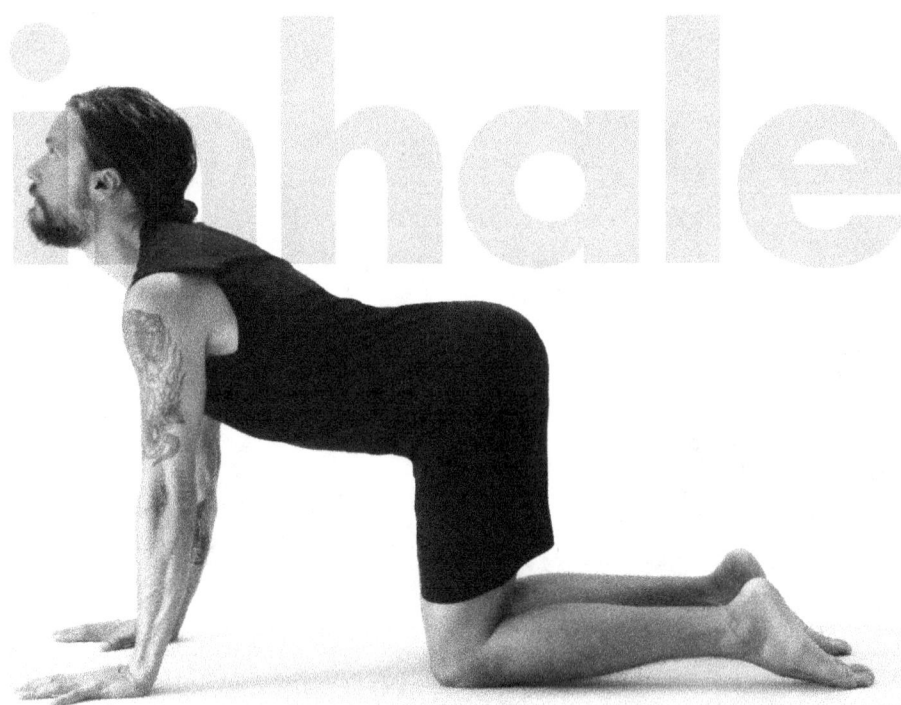

Getting there: Following the instructions on pages 84-85, find your way to your hands and knees, weight equally balanced and spine long.

Inhale as you lift your head and allow your belly to relax, creating an arch in your back. Focus the inhalation in your chest.

exhale

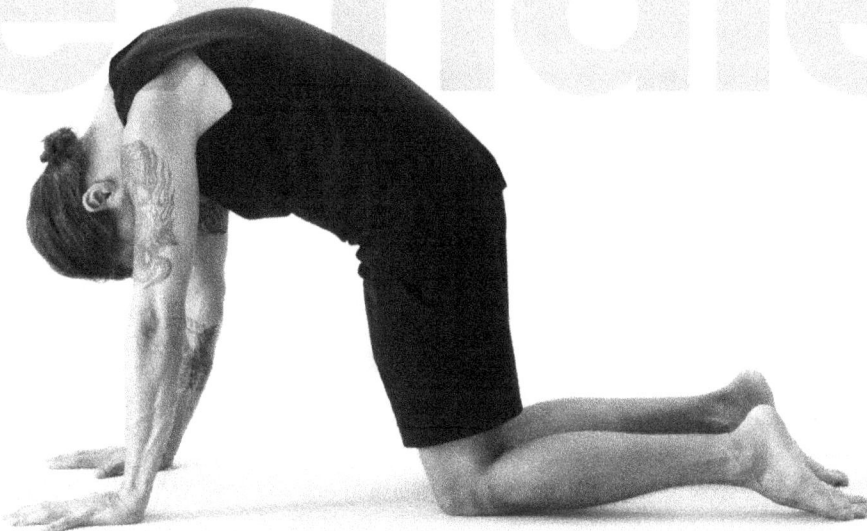

Exhale as you drop your head and tailbone, lifting your mid-back toward the sky. Draw your belly up and in as you exhale. <u>Repeat</u> the movement a number of times.

deep crouch

inhale

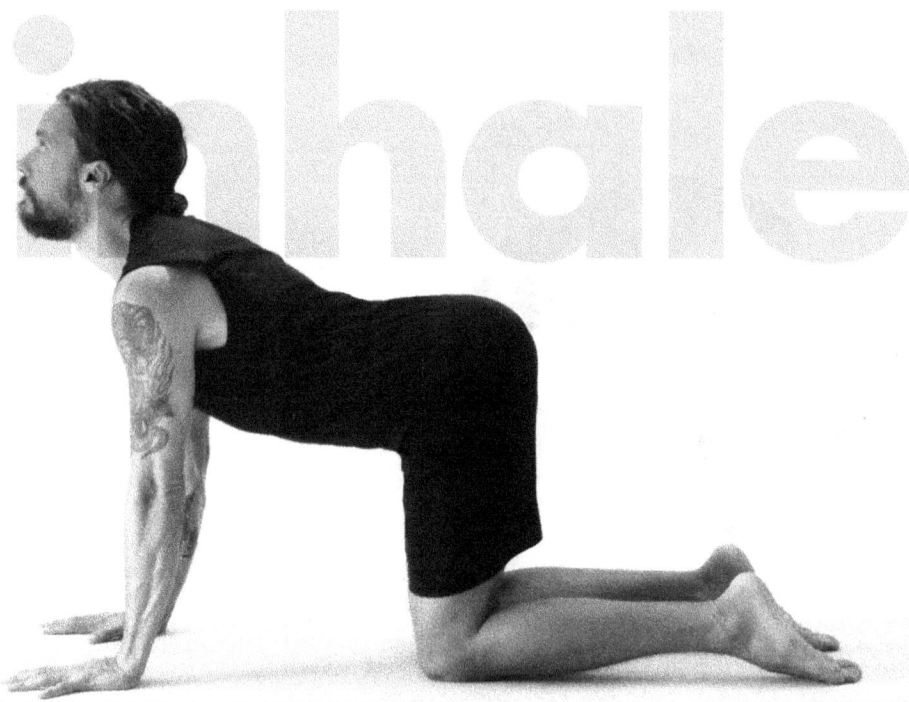

Inhale as you lift your head and allow your belly to relax, creating an arch in your back. Focus the inhalation in your chest.

exhale

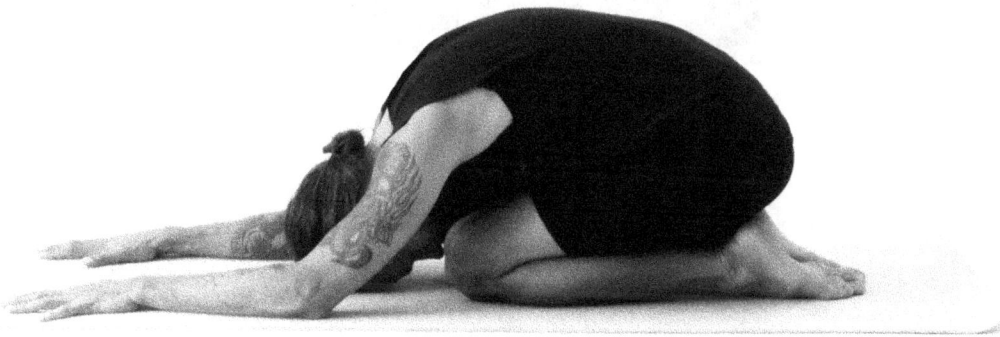

Exhale as you push your hips back and down toward your heels, eventually resting your forehead on the ground, arms relaxed. <u>Repeat</u> the movement a number of times.

leg extension

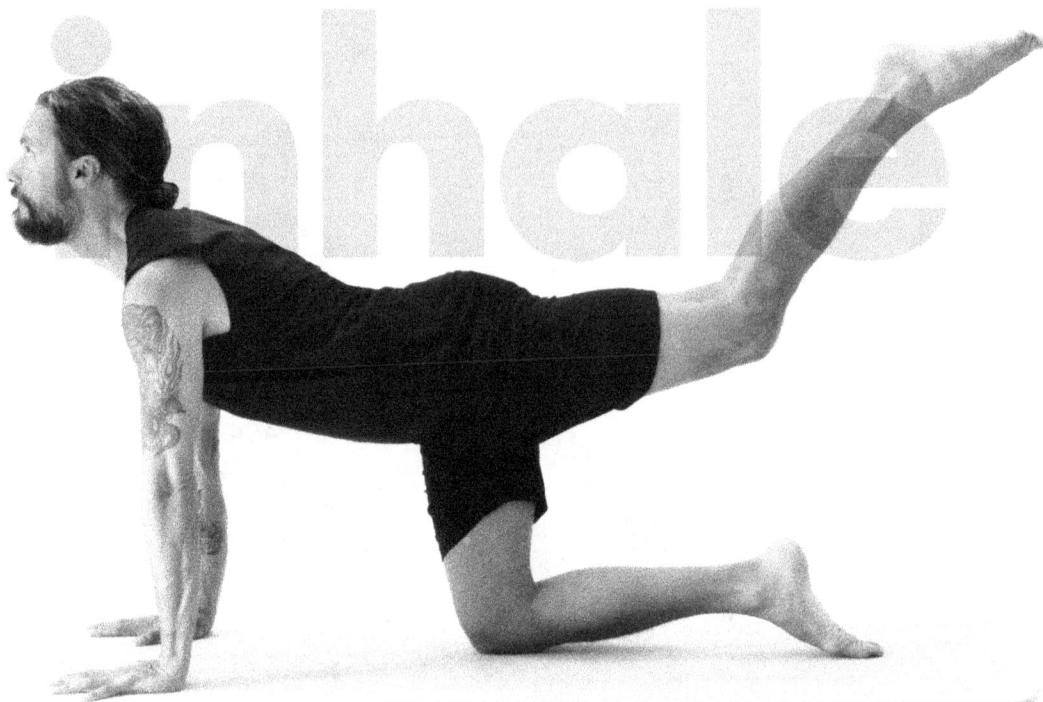

Inhale as you lift your head and one leg, creating an arch in your back. Engage your backside muscles to support the leg lift. Focus the inhalation in your chest and pause in this position.

exhale

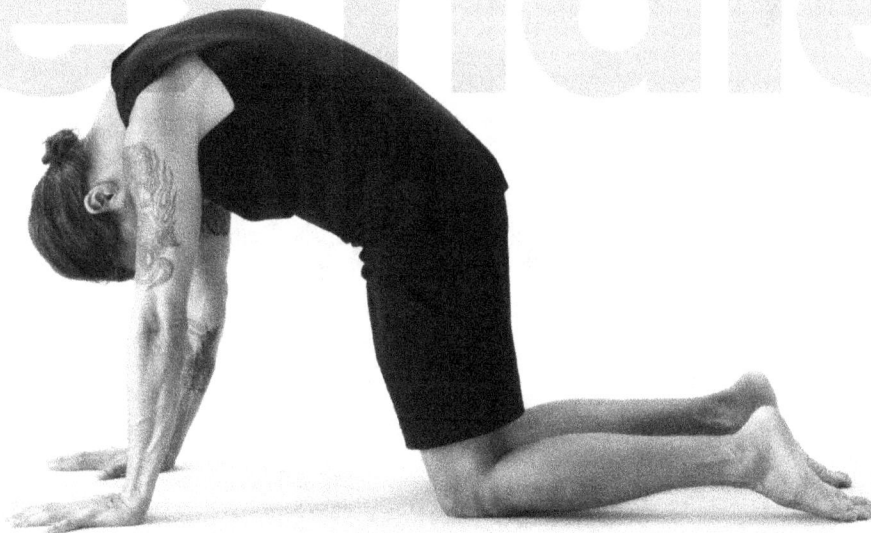

Exhale as you return your knee to the ground and drop your head and tailbone, lifting your mid-back toward the sky. Draw your belly up and in as you exhale. <u>Repeat</u> the movement a number of times lifting alternating legs on inhale. <u>Stay</u> in the 'inhale' position for an equal amount of time on each side. <u>Intensify</u> the movement by drawing your knee in toward your chest on exhalation. Repeat a number of times, then switch sides.

leg & arm extension

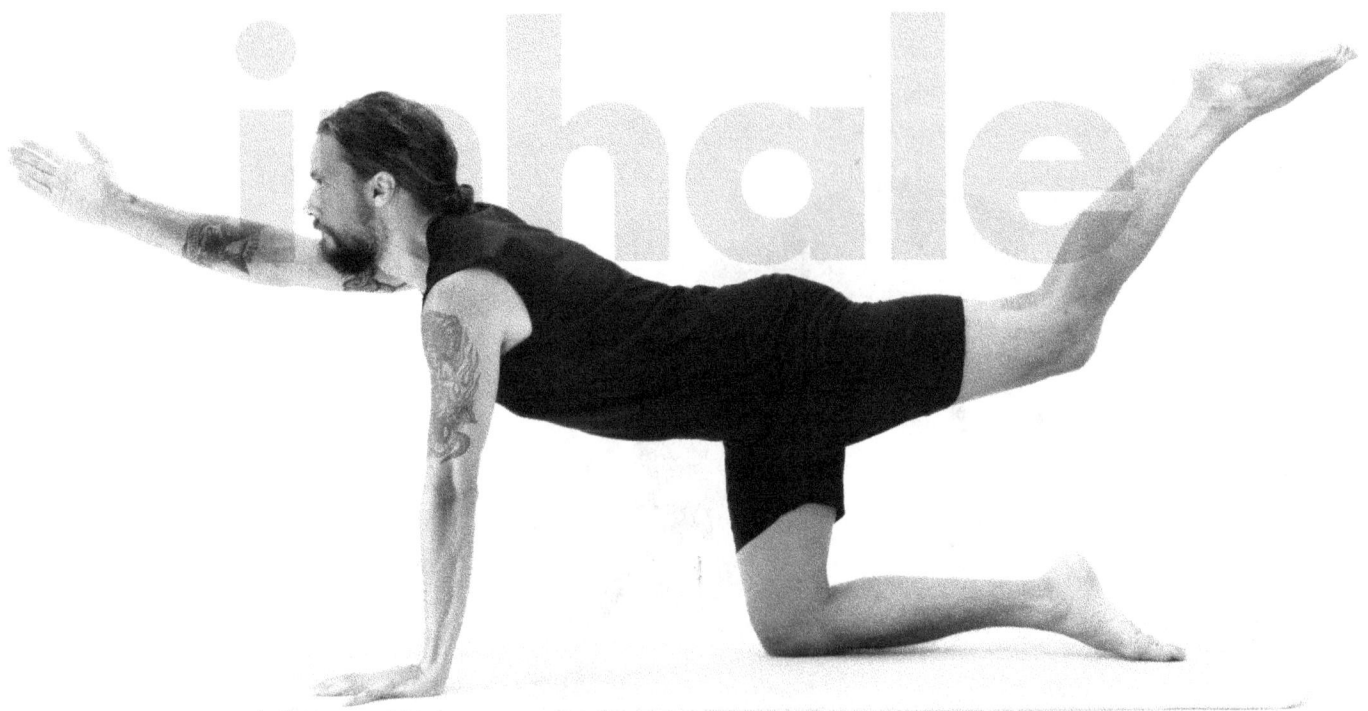

Inhale as you lift one leg and the opposite arm, creating an arch in your back. Pause in this position, engaging your backside muscles for support.

exhale

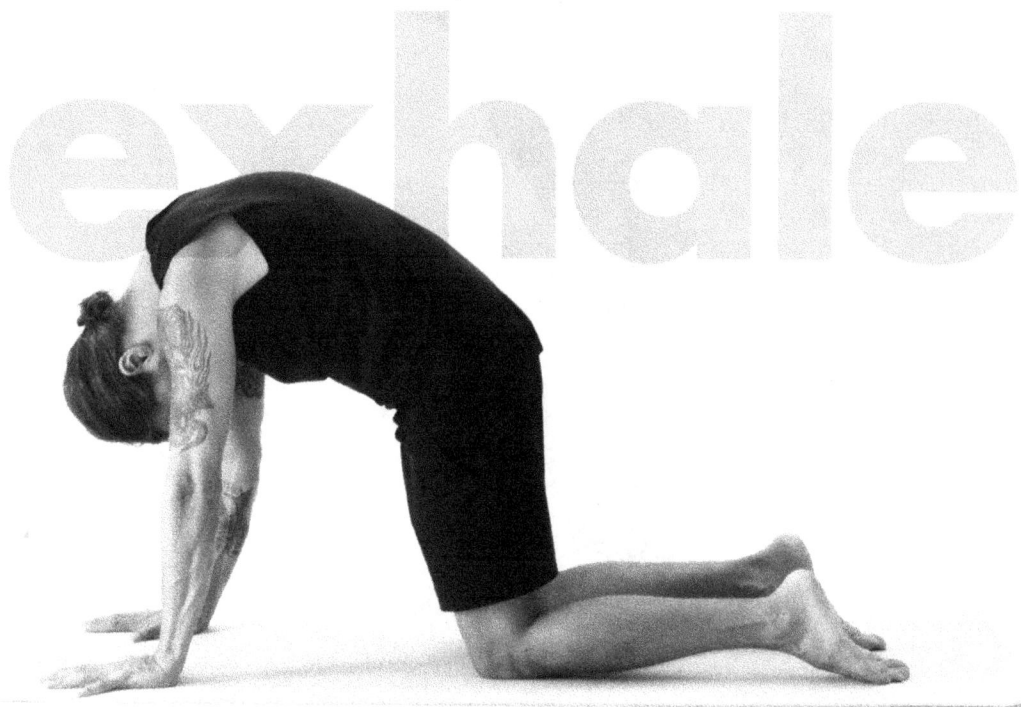

Exhale as you return your hand and knee to the ground, dropping your head and tailbone, lifting your mid-back toward the sky. Draw your belly up and in as you exhale. <u>Repeat</u> the movement a number of times alternating sides on each inhalation. <u>Stay</u> in the 'inhale' position for an equal amount of time on each side.

kneeling forward bend

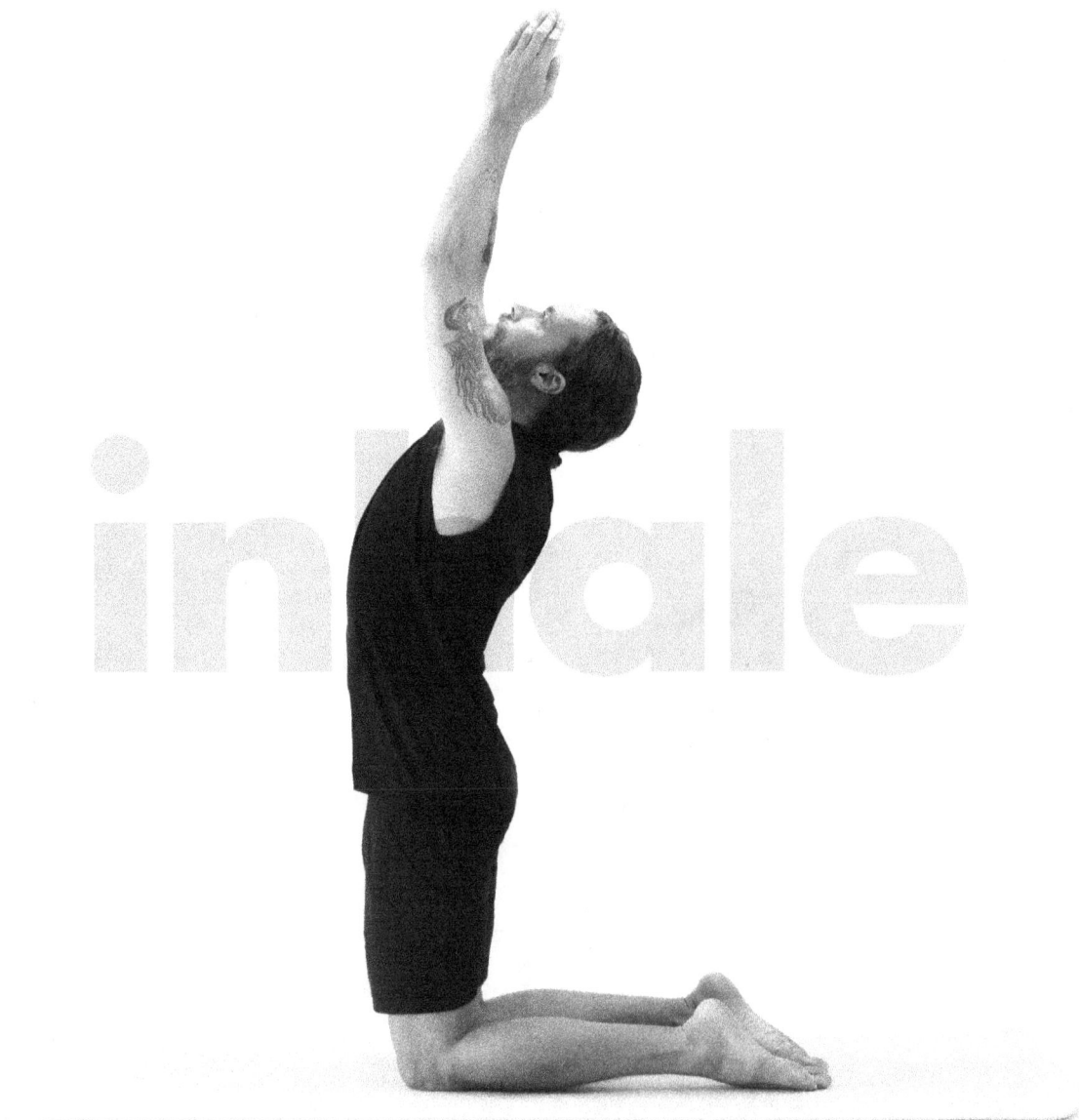

Getting there: Start in a deep kneeling crouch position, with your hands resting on your lower back, palms turned up and forehead on the ground (this is the exhale position).
Inhale as you stand up on your knees and sweep your arms overhead. Look up and see your hands come together. Engage your backside muscles.

exhale

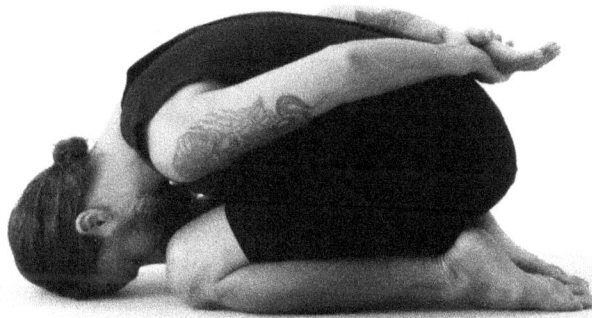

Exhale as you sit back on your heels, simultaneously returning your hands to your lower back. Rest your forehead on the ground. <u>Repeat</u> the movement a number of times.

kneeling arm raises

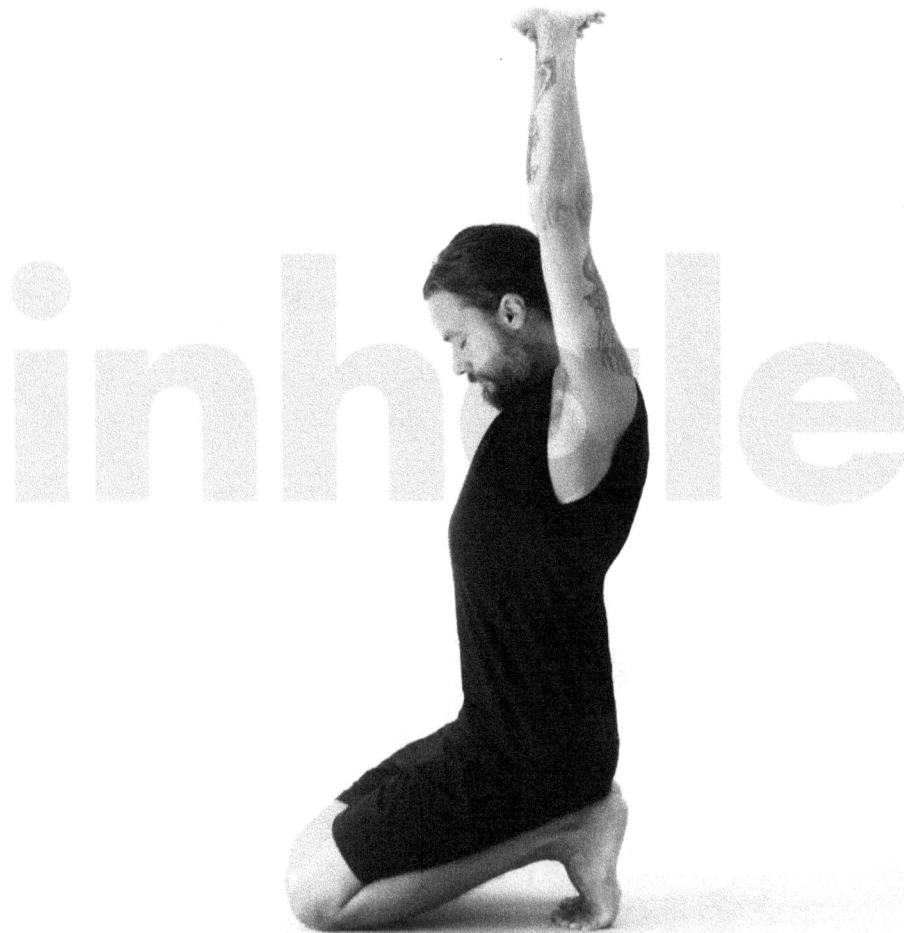

Getting there: Start in a kneeling position with your toes curled under, stretching the bottoms of your feet. Interlace your fingers behind your head.
Inhale as you straighten your arms, palms toward the sky. Keep your chin lowered to your chest throughout the entire movement.

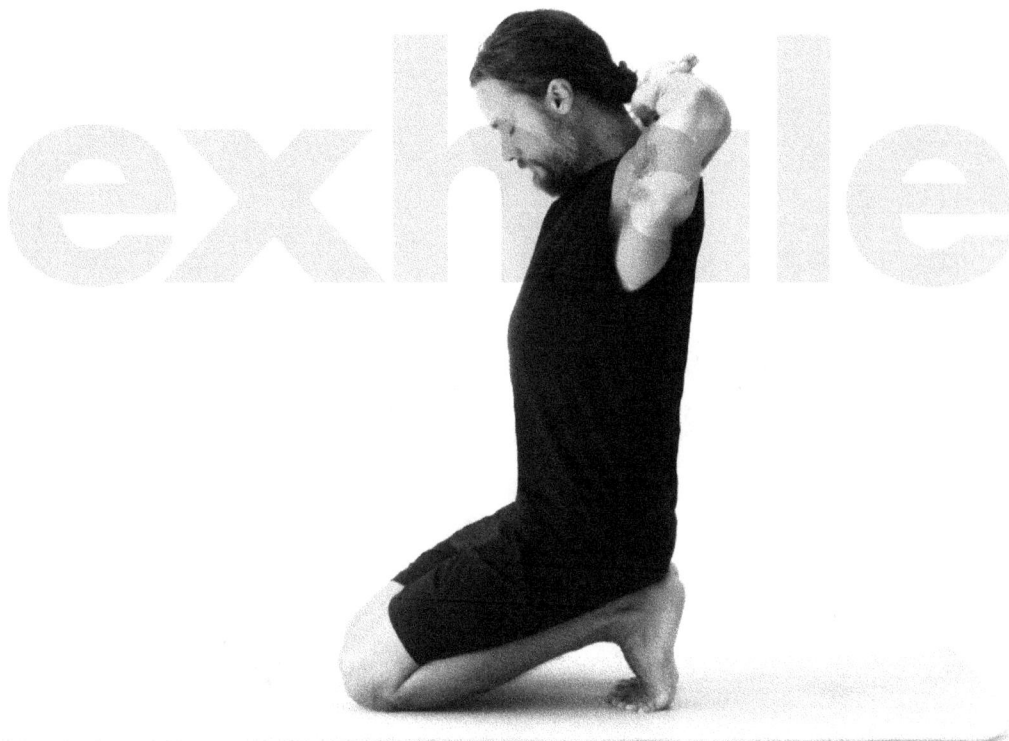

Exhale as you bend your elbows and squeeze your shoulderblades together. Pause and draw your elbows back, opening your chest a little more. Repeat the movement a number of times. Variation: Repeat this same movement with your toes untucked, stretching the tops of your feet.

lunging shoulder sweep

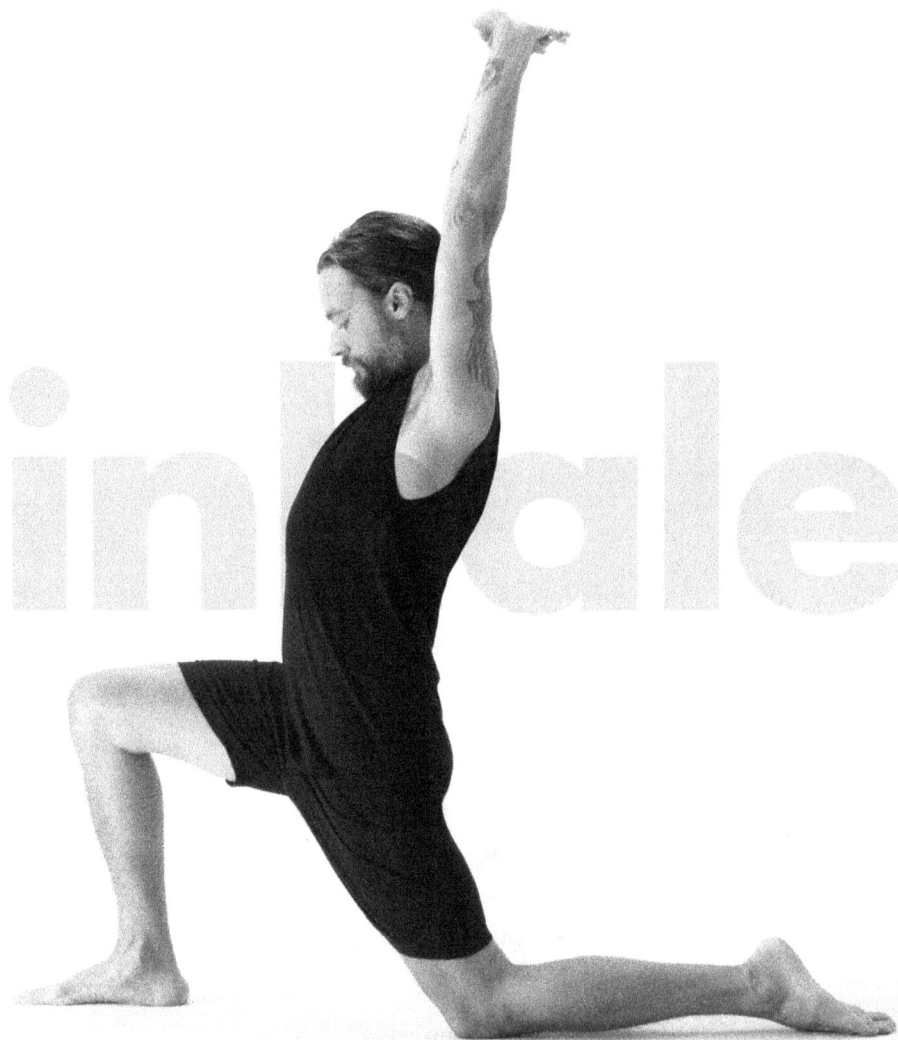

Getting there: Start standing on your knees with your toes untucked, and bring one leg out in front, knee bent to about 90°. Interlace your fingers behind your head.

Inhale as you straighten your arms toward the sky. Keep your chin lowered. Pause and feel the stretch in the front of your hip.

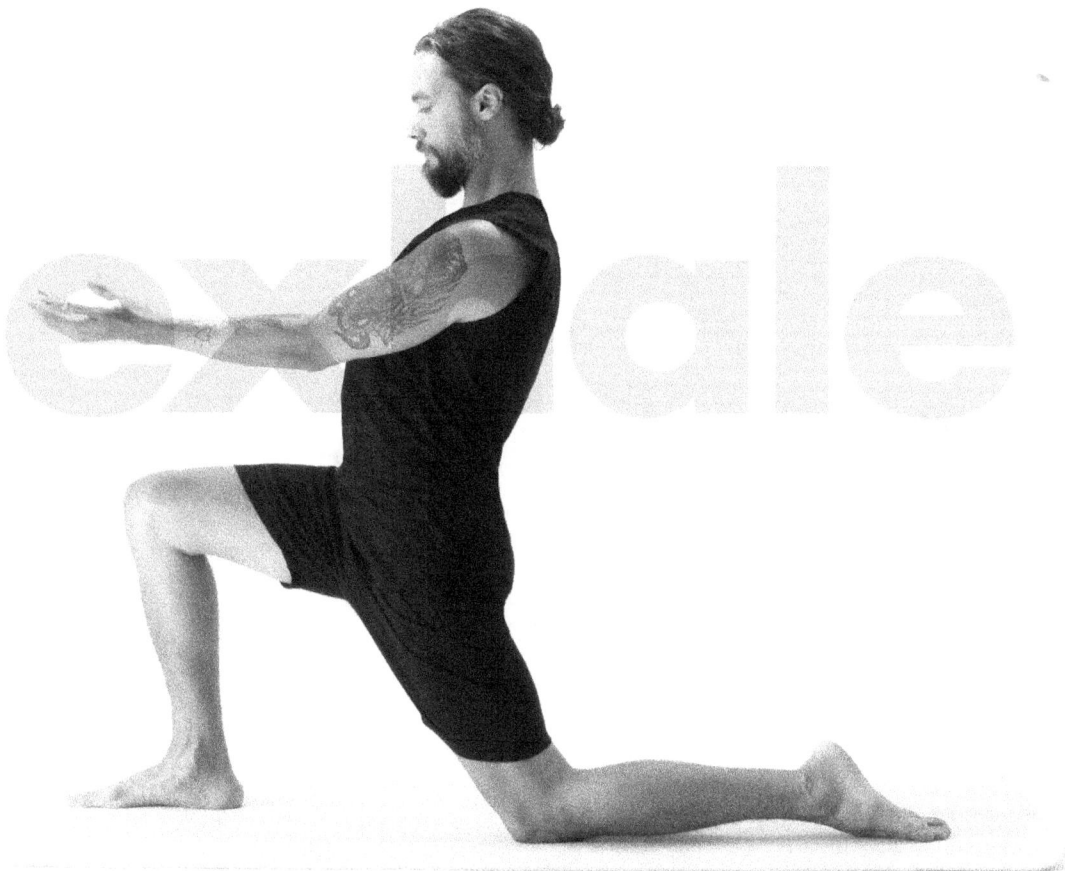

Exhale as you sweep your arms in a wide circle, bringing your hands in front of you, palms turned up. <u>Repeat</u> the movement a number of times. Switch the forward leg and repeat the entire sequence.

3.4 seated & supine movements

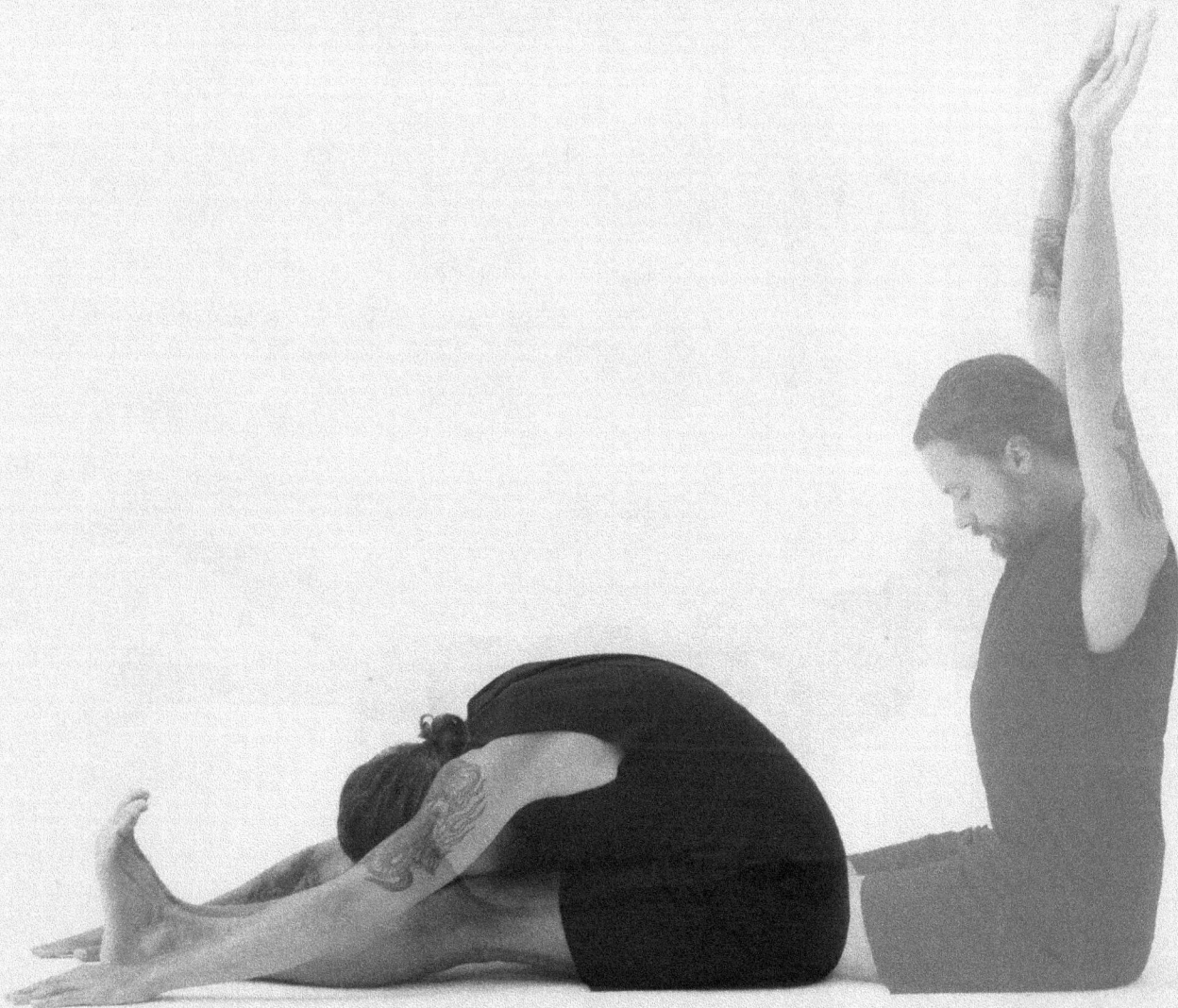

leg & arm lift

inhale

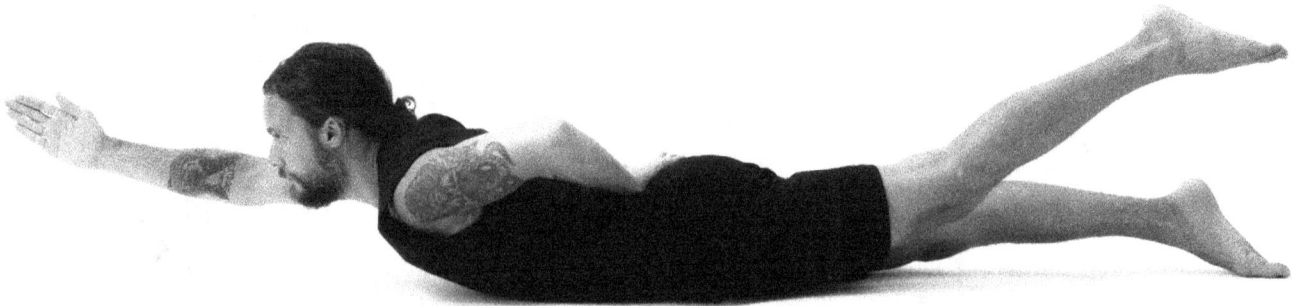

Getting there: Start by lying on your stomach, legs together and stretched out, palms turned up and resting on your lower back (this is the exhale position).
Inhale as you lift one arm and the opposite leg, lifting your chest and head. Look at your outstretched hand.

exhale

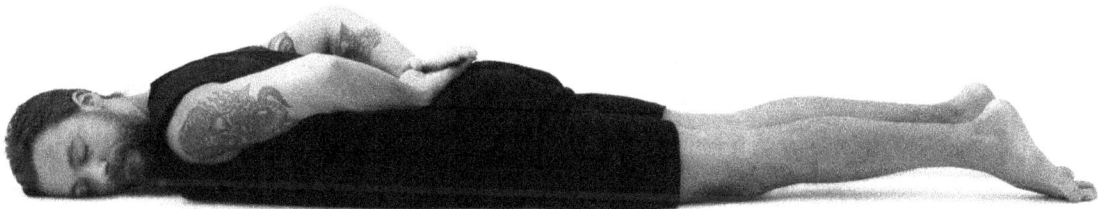

Exhale as you return your leg to the ground and your outstretched hand to your lower back. Lower your head, turning it to rest on one side. <u>Repeat</u> the movement, alternating the lifting leg and arm on inhale, and turning your head to rest on the other side.

full back extension

inhale

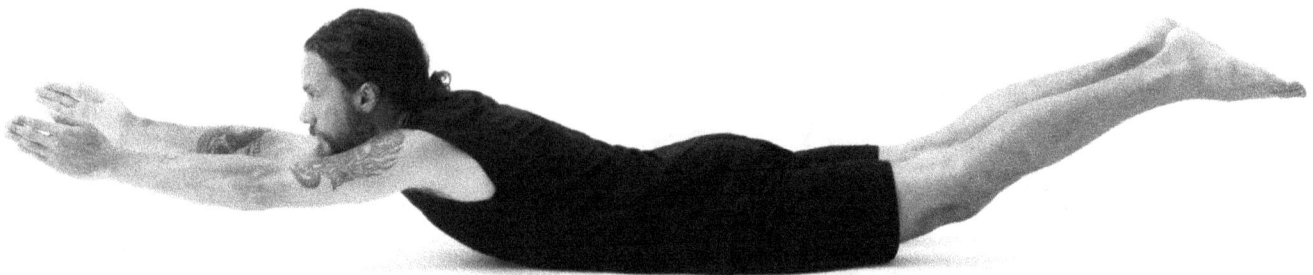

Getting there: Start by lying on your stomach, legs together and stretched out, palms turned up and resting on your lower back (this is the exhale position).
Inhale as you sweep both arms out in front, both legs lifting off the ground, at the same time lifting your head and chest.

exhale

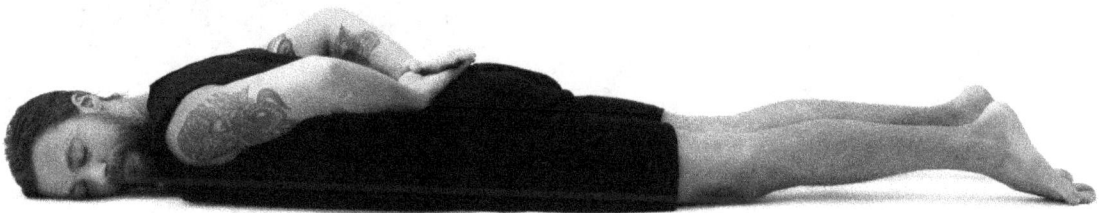

Exhale as you return your legs to the ground and your hands to your lower back. Turn and lower your head, resting on your cheek. Repeat the sequence a number of times, turning your head to alternating sides on exhalation. Stay in the 'inhale' position for a number of breaths.

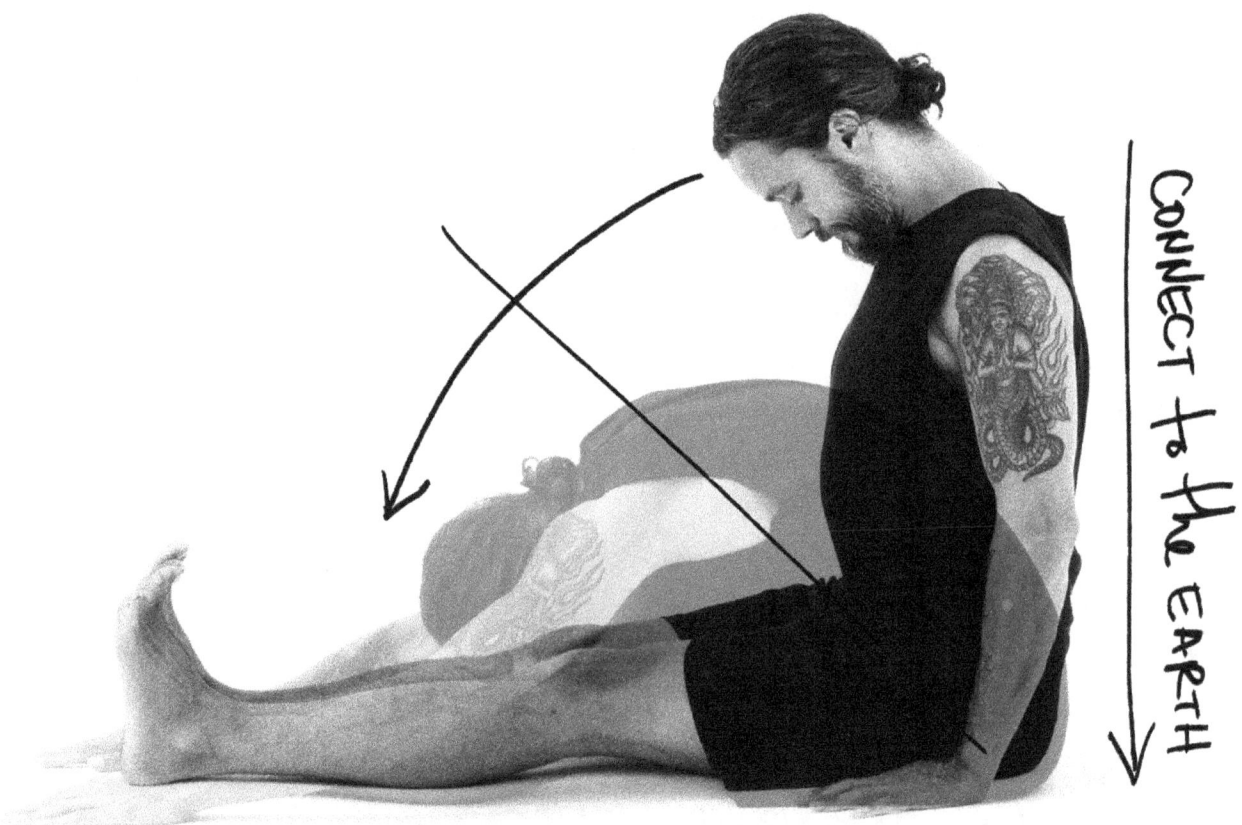

CONNECT to the EARTH

find the ground.

Connect to the earth through your sitting bones. Let that connection be the foundation for your movement.

seated forward bend

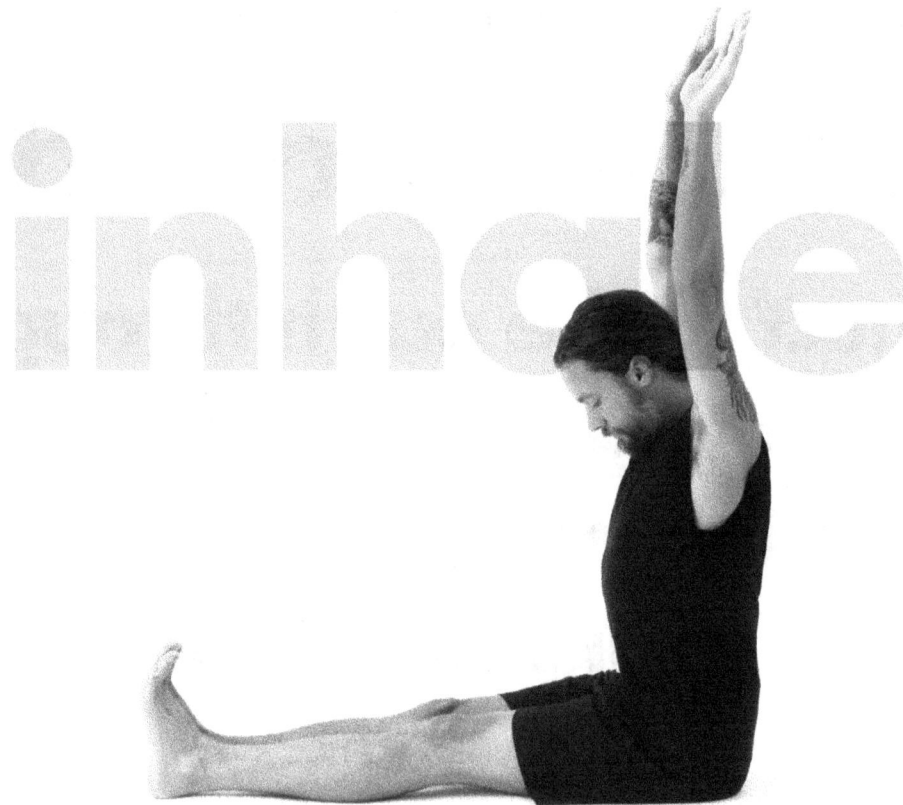

inhale

Getting there: Start by sitting with your legs stretched out in front and your torso upright. **Inhale** as you lift both arms straight up and overhead, keeping your chin down. <u>Modify</u> by bending your knees or placing a rolled up blanket or towel under them for support. Try to avoid rounding your lower back.

exhale

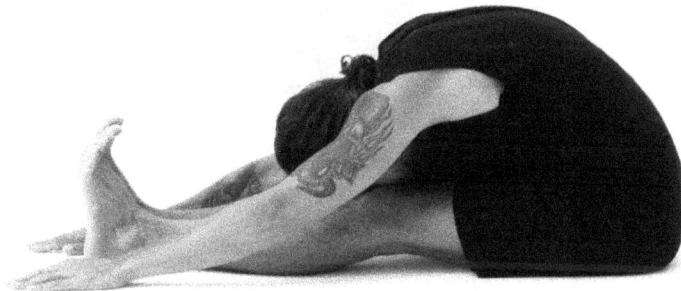

Exhale as you hinge at the waist, and keep your arms extended until you complete the forward bend. If you feel a strain in the back of your legs, modify by bending your knees. Note the difference between 'stretch' and 'strain'. <u>Repeat</u> the movement a number of times. <u>Stay</u> in the 'exhale' position for a number of breaths.

head-to-knee

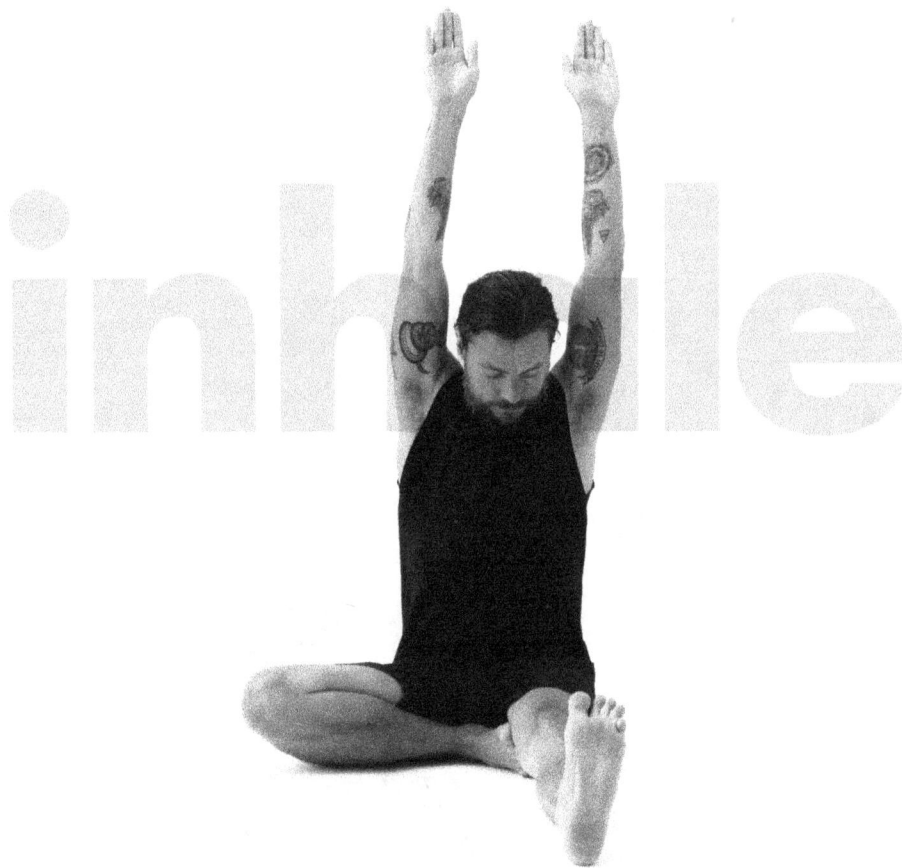

Getting there: Start by sitting with your legs stretched out in front and your torso upright (see previous spread). Take one foot in as close to your groin as you comfortably can resting the sole of your foot on the inside of the extended leg.

Inhale as you lift both arms straight up and overhead, keeping your chin down.

exhale

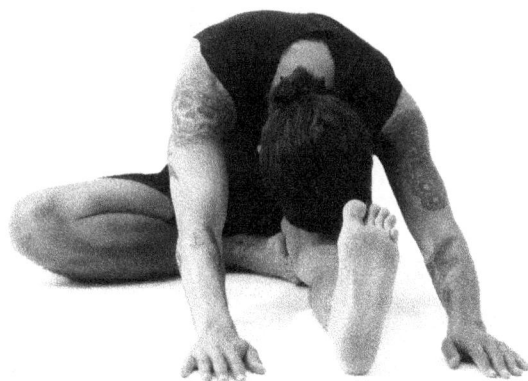

Exhale as you hinge forward at the waist, keeping your arms extended until you complete the forward bend. If you feel a strain in your outstretched leg, bend your knee or place a rolled-up towel under it. <u>Repeat</u> the movement a number of times. <u>Stay</u> in the 'exhale' position for a number of breaths, then switch legs and repeat the entire sequence.

side straddle

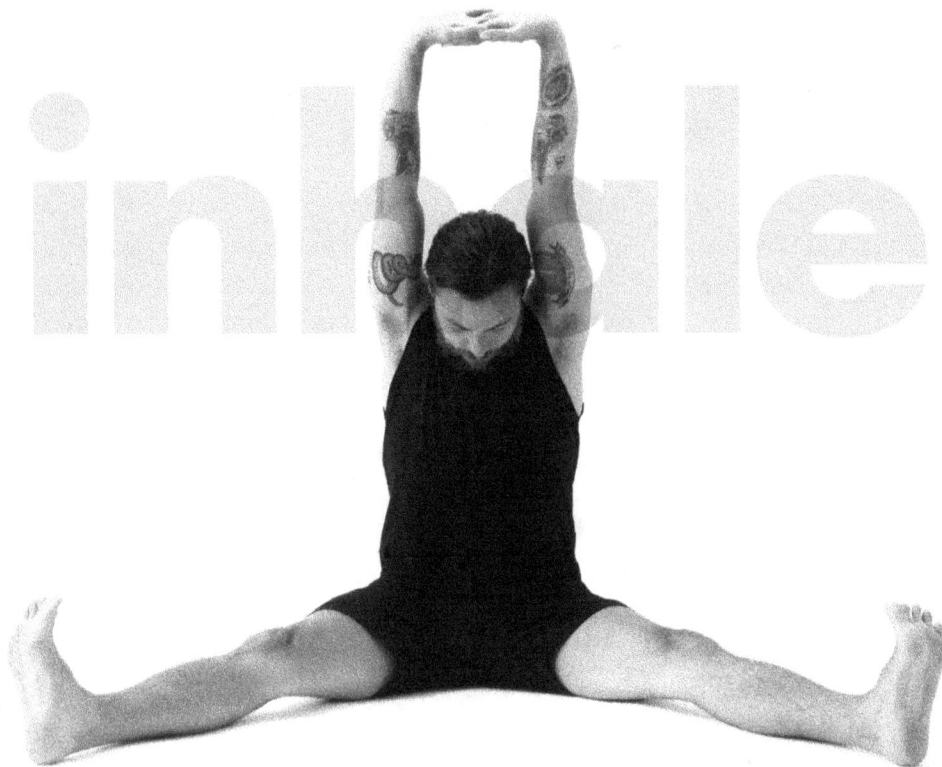

Getting there: Start by sitting with your legs stretched out in front and open to about a 90° angle. Keep your legs and feet active.

Inhale as you lift both arms straight up and overhead. Interlace your fingers and keep your chin lowered. <u>Modify</u> by bending your knees if you're unable to sit upright without your lower back rounding.

exhale

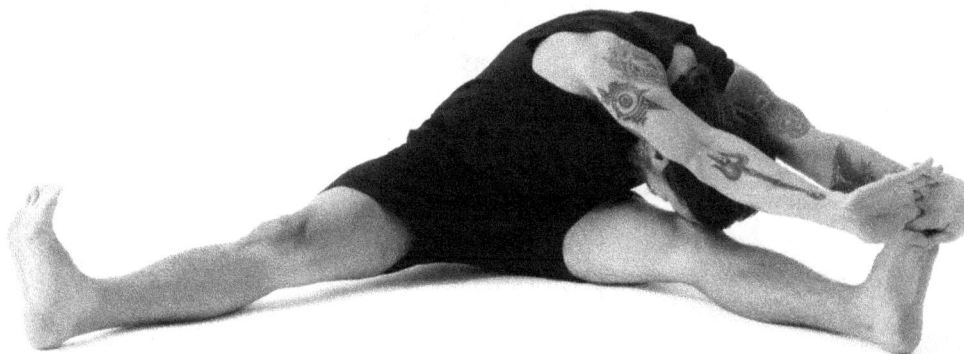

Exhale as you turn and bend toward one leg, keeping your arms outstretched and spine long. You should feel a slight twist in your lower back but no straining. Repeat the movement a number of times, alternating sides every exhalation. Stay in the 'exhale' position for an equal amount of time on each side.

straddle

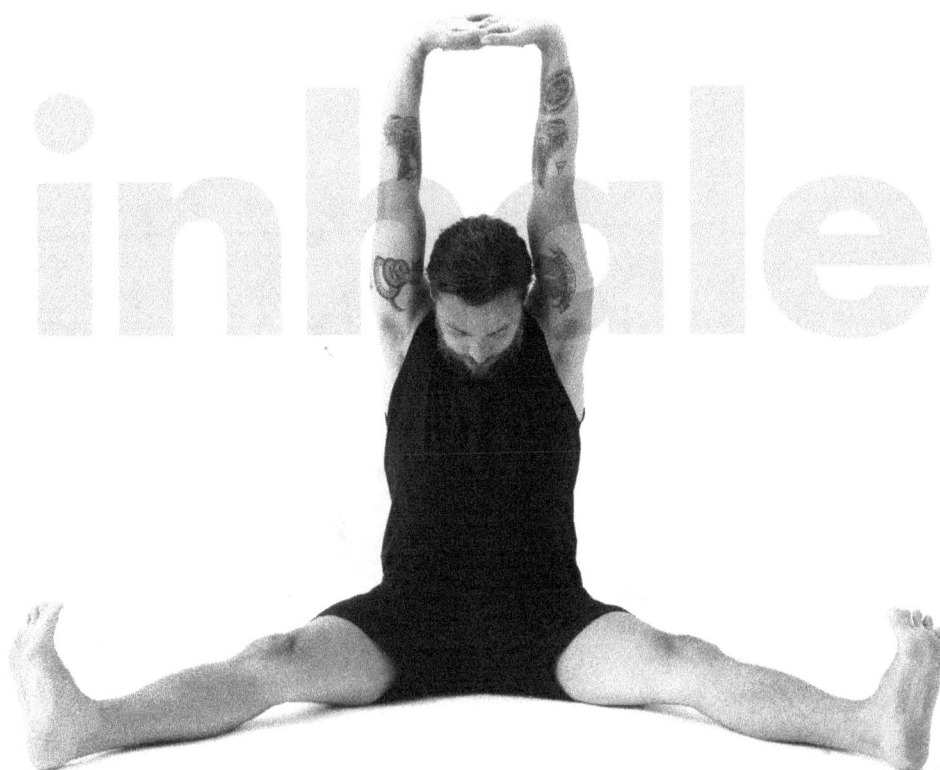

Getting there: Start by sitting with your legs stretched out in front and open to about a 90°
angle. Keep your legs and feet active.
Inhale as you lift both arms straight up and overhead. Interlace your fingers and keep your chin
lowered. <u>Modify</u> by bending your knees if you can't sit upright without your lower back rounding.

exhale

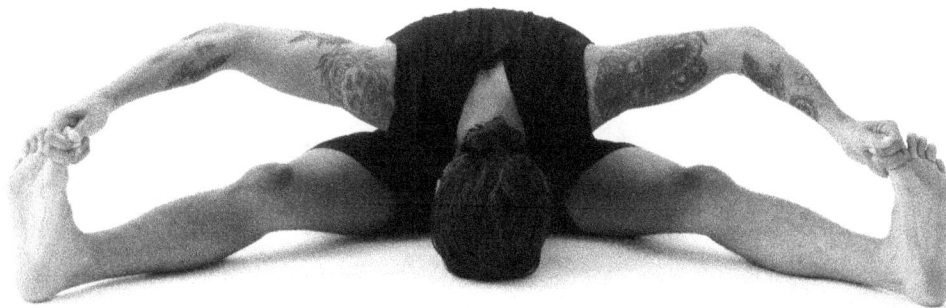

Exhale as you hinge at the waist, bending forward and keeping your arms outstretched. Stay in the 'exhale' position for a number of breaths. Try this: When you stay in the 'exhale' position, grasp your big toes with your first two fingers and thumb. Pull up to help lengthen your spine forward.

single leg lift

inhale

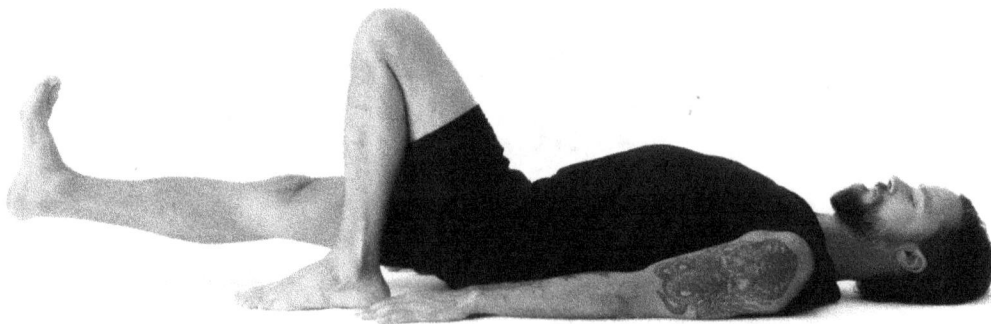

Getting there: Start by lying down on your back with your legs together and stretched out, arms at your side. Bend one leg and place that foot close to your hip. Activate the straight leg. **Inhale** as you lift the extended leg until it's just above the ground. On each subsequent inhalation, you'll return your leg to this starting position, hovering just above the ground.

exhale

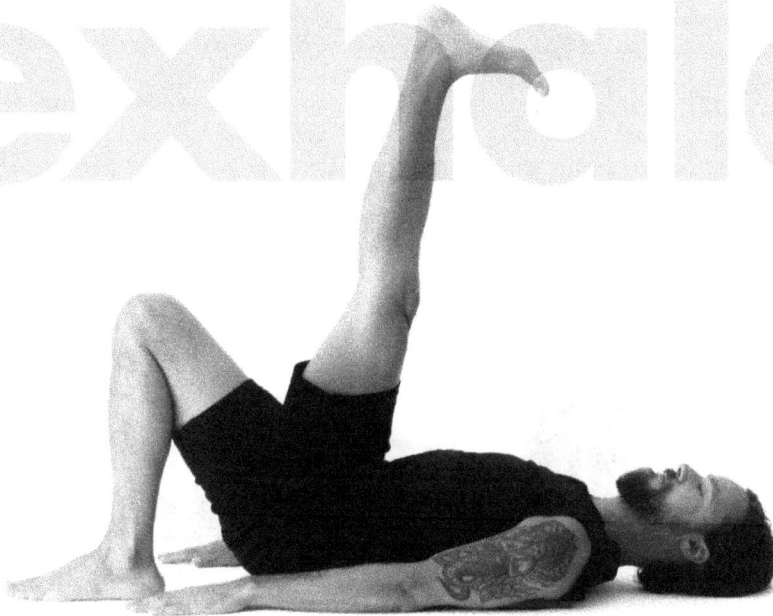

Exhale as you lift the extended leg as high as you can while keeping it straight. <u>Repeat</u> the movement a number of times, inhale lower, exhale lift. Switch legs and repeat the sequence an equal number of times.Intensify the movement by keeping the stationary leg straight throughout.

single leg lift with arms

inhale

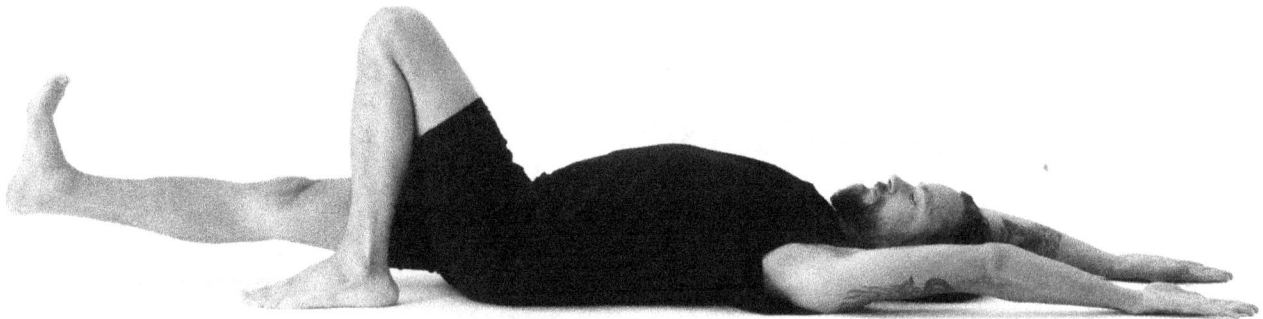

Getting there: Start by lying down on your back with your legs together and stretched out, arms at your side. Bend one leg and place that foot close to your hip.

Inhale as you bring both arms overhead, and lift the extended leg until it's just above the ground. On each subsequent inhalation, you'll return your leg to this starting position, hovering just above the ground with your arms stretched overhead.

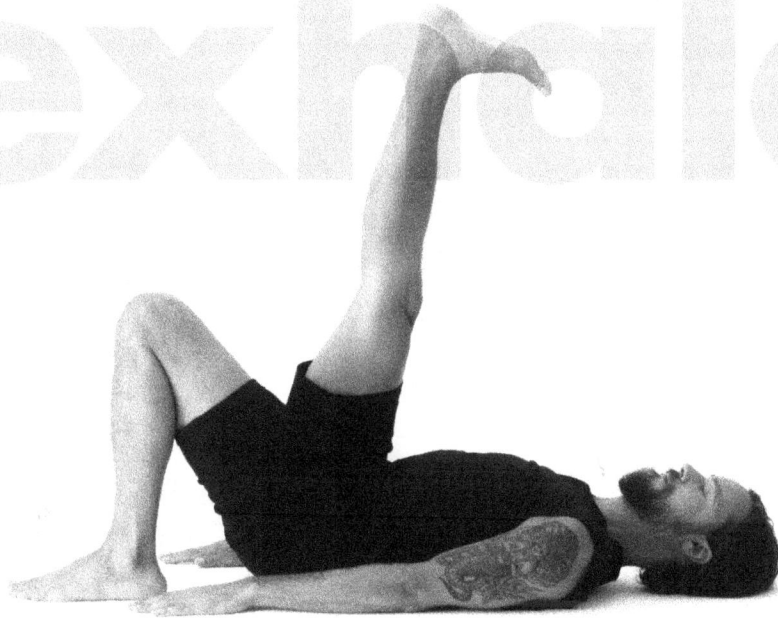

Exhale as you lift the extended leg as high as you can while keeping it straight, at the same time bringing your arms to your side. Repeat the movement a number of times. Inhale lower, exhale lift. Switch legs and repeat the sequence an equal number of times. Intensify the movement by keeping the stationary leg straight throughout.

double leg lift

inhale

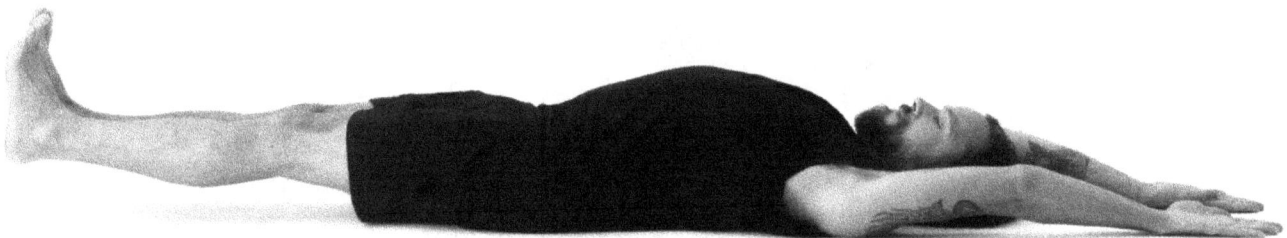

Getting there: Start by lying down on your back with your legs together and stretched out, arms at your side. <u>Inhale</u> as you lift both arms overhead, lifting both legs just above the ground. Keep your feet together.

exhale

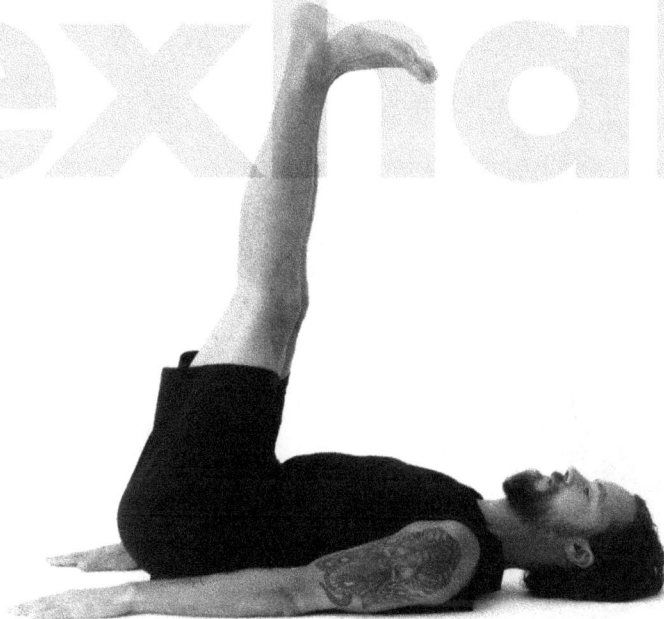

Exhale as you lift both legs as high as you can while keeping them straight, at the same time bringing your arms down to your side. <u>Repeat</u> the movement a number of times, pausing for a moment after exhalation as you contract your abdominals. Inhale lower your legs, exhale lift them. <u>Stay</u> in the 'exhale' position for a number of breaths.

legs to the sky

inhale

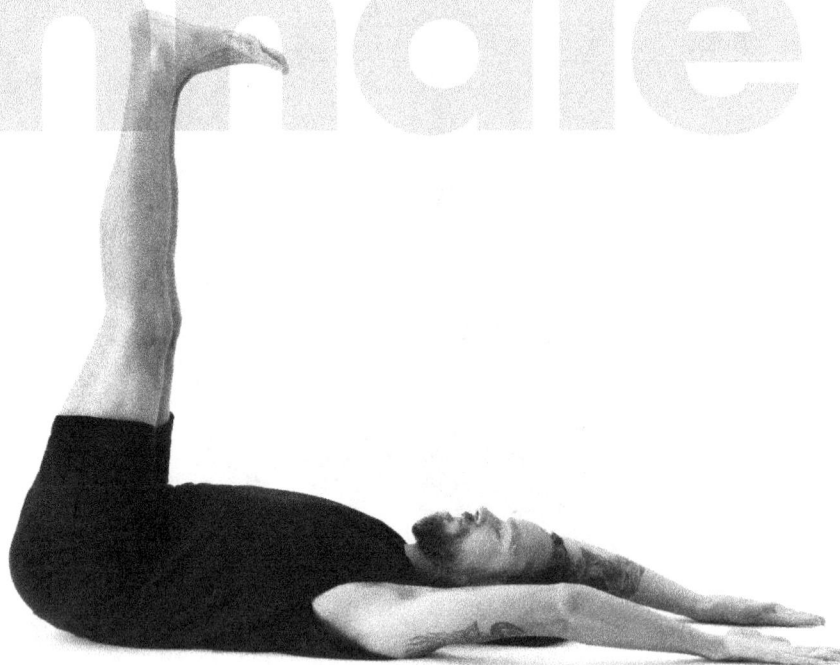

Getting there: Start by lying down on your back with your legs bent toward your chest and your hands resting on your knees or shins.

Inhale as you lift both arms overhead, raising and straightening both legs toward the sky to make an 'L' shape.

exhale

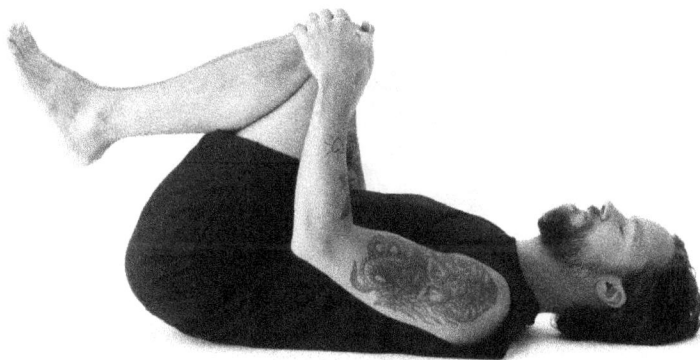

Exhale as you contract your abdominals and bend both legs, knees toward your chest and a hand on each knee. <u>Repeat</u> the movement a number of times. <u>Stay</u> in the 'inhale' position for a number of breaths. <u>Try this</u>: while performing the movements, hold your breath for 2 seconds after both the inhalation and exhalation.

inverted straddle

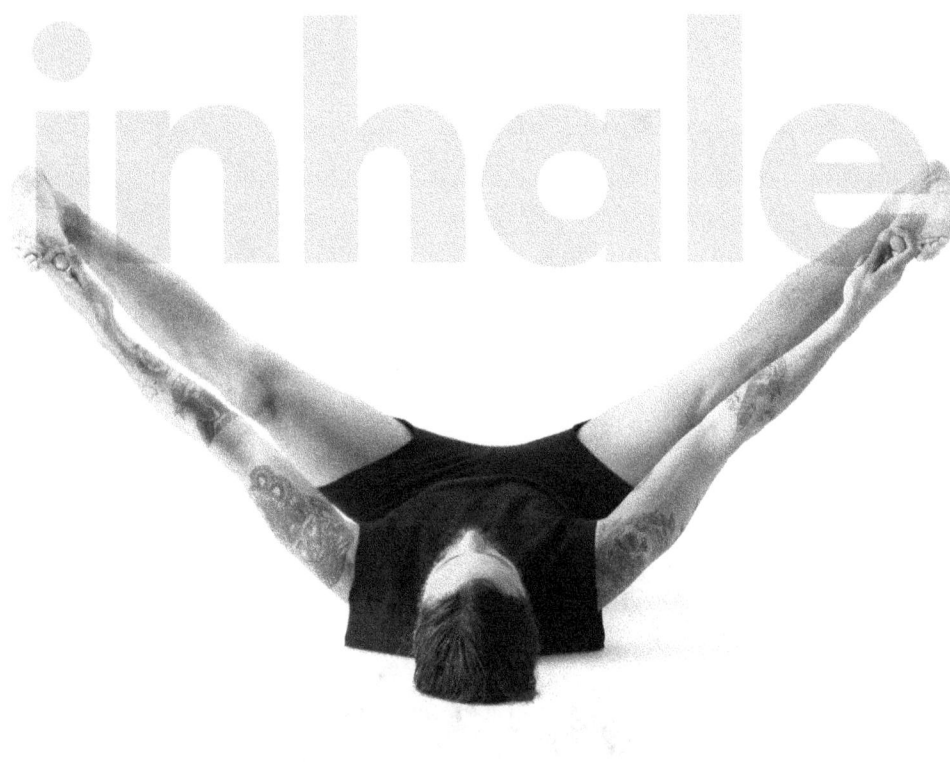

Getting there: Start by lying down on your back with your legs lifted, grasping your big toes with your first two fingers and thumb. If needed, bend your knees a little.

Inhale as you open your legs in a 'V' shape. <u>Modify</u> by holding your outer thighs if you can't reach your toes and perform the movement.

exhale

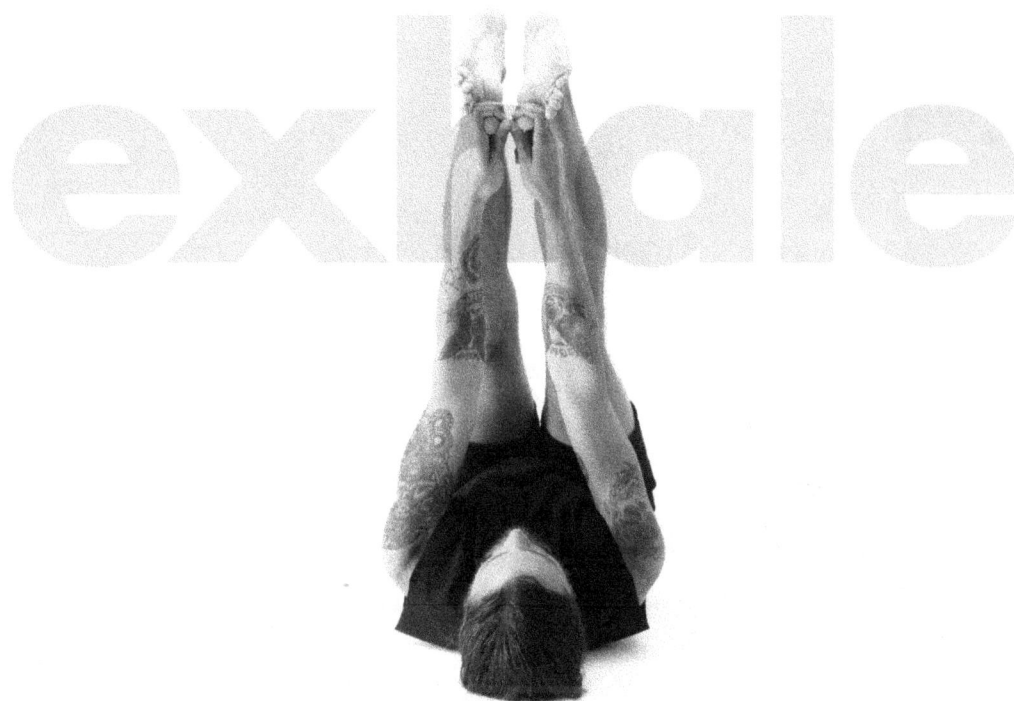

Exhale as you bring your legs together, holding your toes. <u>Repeat</u> the movement a number of times. <u>Stay</u> in the 'inhale' position for a number of breaths.

half bridge

inhale

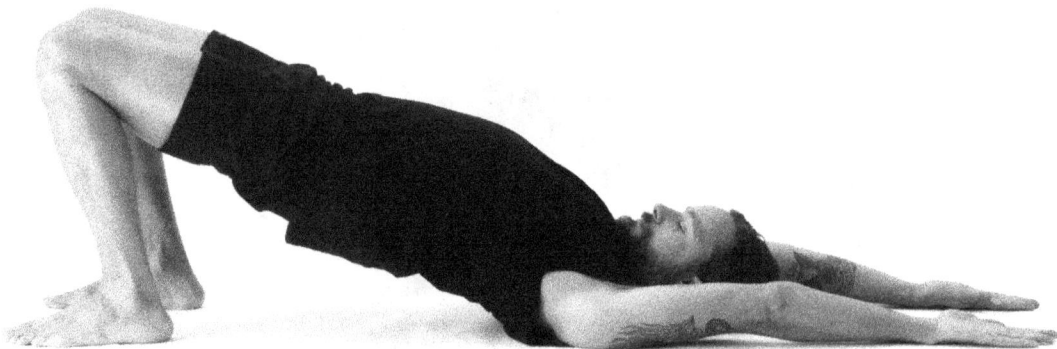

Getting there: Start by lying down on your back with your legs bent and feet close to your backside and hip width.

Inhale as you lift both arms overhead, raising your hips toward the sky. Modify the movement if you feel neck strain by keeping your arms at your side.

exhale

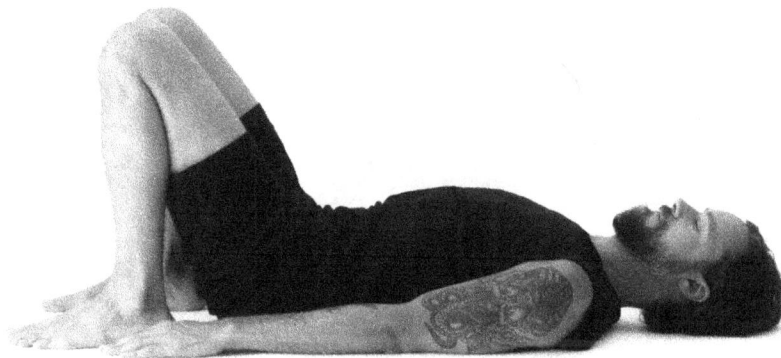

Exhale as you lower your hips to the ground and arms to your side. <u>Repeat</u> the movement a number of times. <u>Stay</u> in the 'inhale' position for a number of breaths.

one-legged bridge

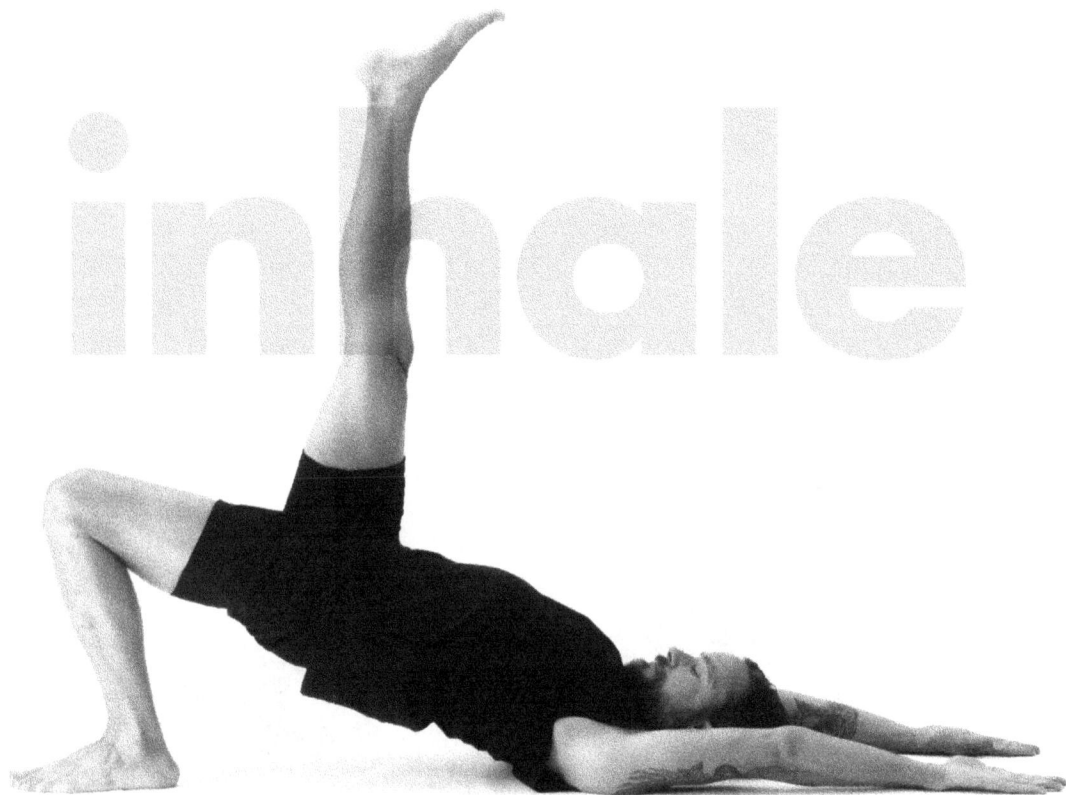

Getting there: Start in the half bridge position shown on the previous spread. **Inhale** as you lift one leg toward the sky, keeping it as straight as you can.

exhale

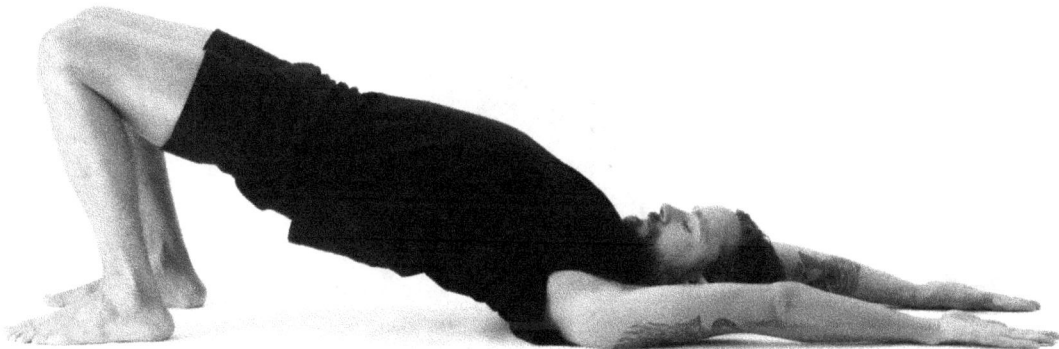

Exhale as you lower the lifted leg, placing your foot back on the ground. Repeat the movement a number of times, lifting alternating legs on inhale. Stay in the 'inhale' position for an equal number of breaths on each side.

abdominal twist

inhale

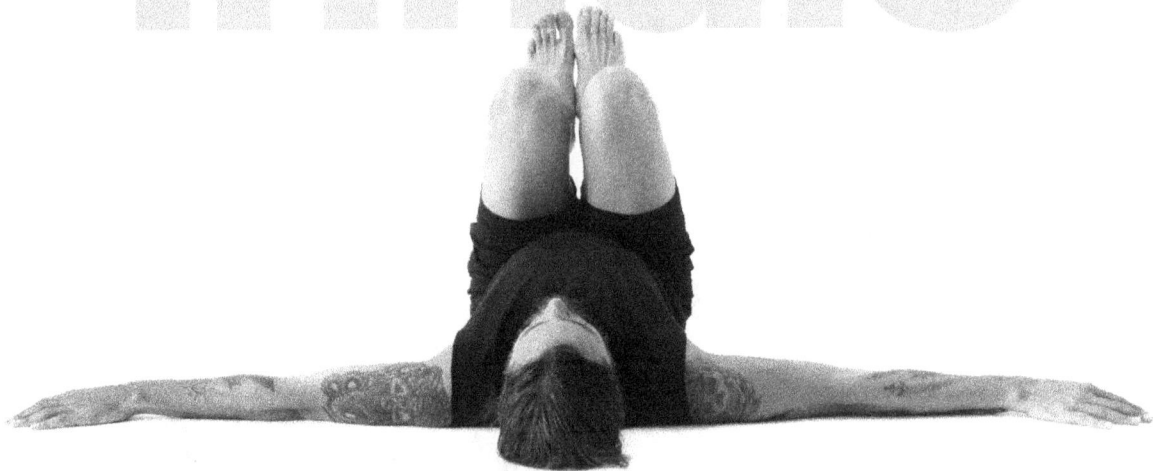

Getting there: Start by lying down on your back with arms outstretched shoulder height, knees bent, feet by your hips.
Inhale as you bring your knees to the center position, keeping them bent and your feet together.

exhale

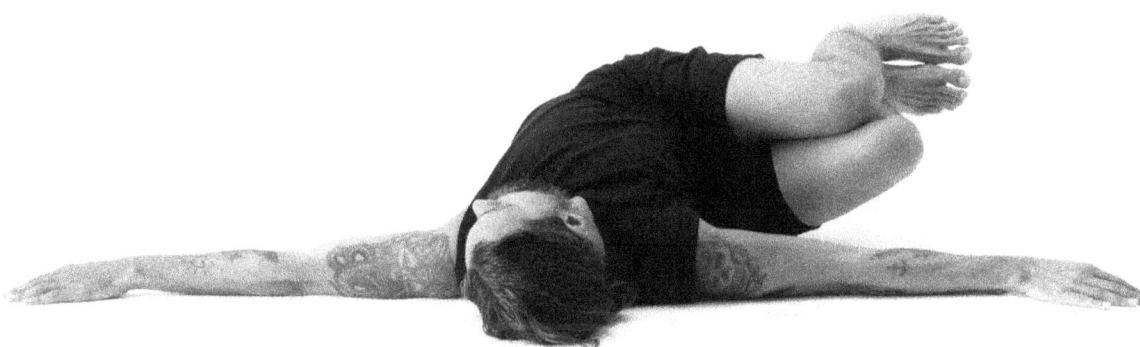

Exhale as you lower both knees to one side. Turn your head in the opposite direction if it's comfortable. <u>Repeat</u> the movement a number of times, alternating sides each exhalation. <u>Stay</u> on each side, allowing your legs to rest on the ground for an equal number of breaths. <u>Modify</u> by keeping your feet on the floor while you perform the twisting movement.

legs up restorative

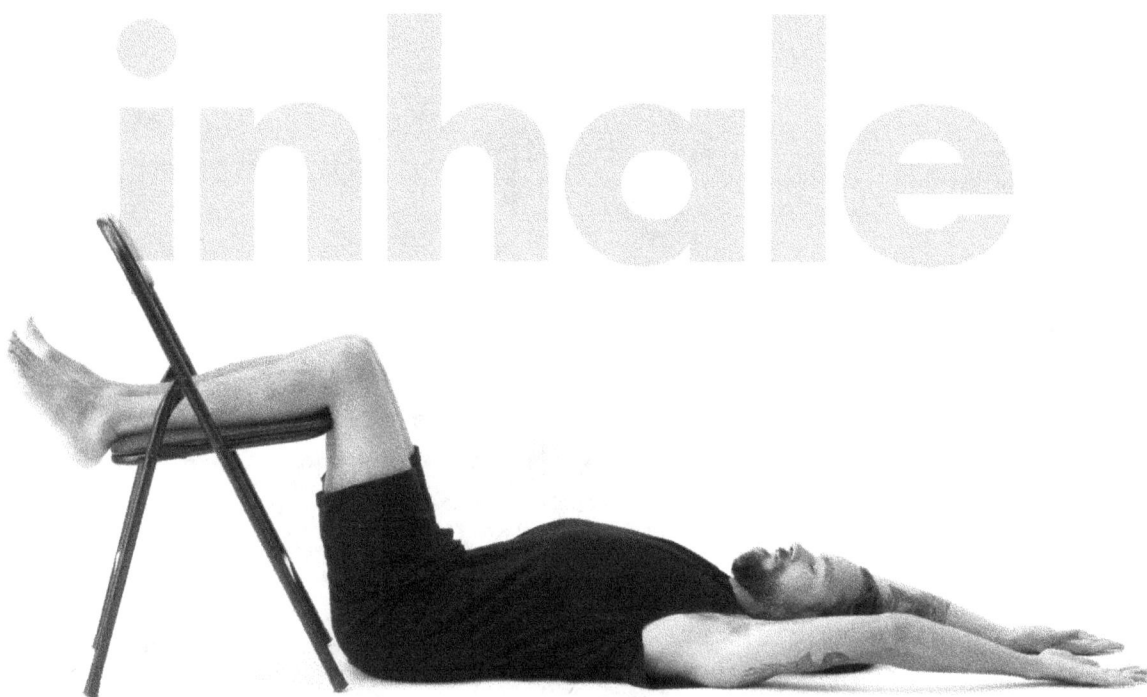

inhale

Getting there: Start by lying down on your back with your legs resting on a chair, arms at your side.

Inhale as you bring your arms straight up overhead, hands to the floor behind or as high as you can comfortably without straining.

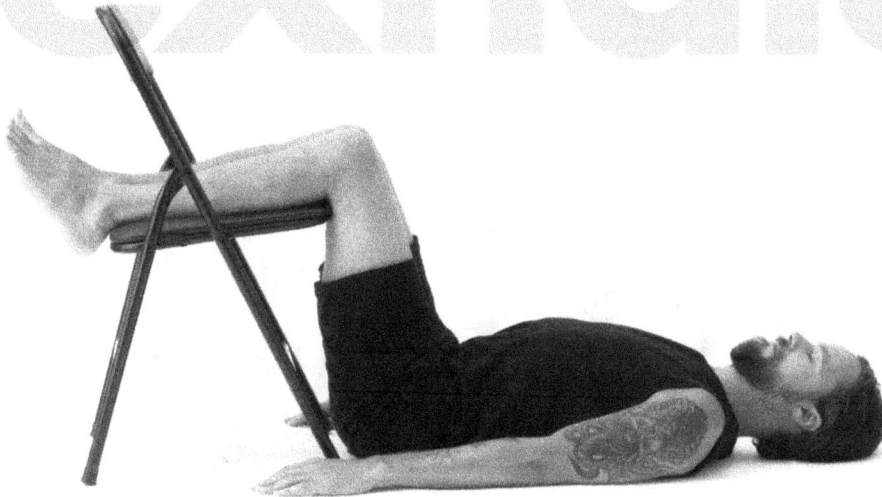

exhale

Exhale as you lower your arms down to your side. <u>Repeat</u> the movement a number of times. <u>Try this</u>: gradually lengthen your exhalation until you are able to maintain a 2:1 breath ratio, exhalation twice as long as inhalation. This may take some time and consistent practice.

bellows breathing

inhale

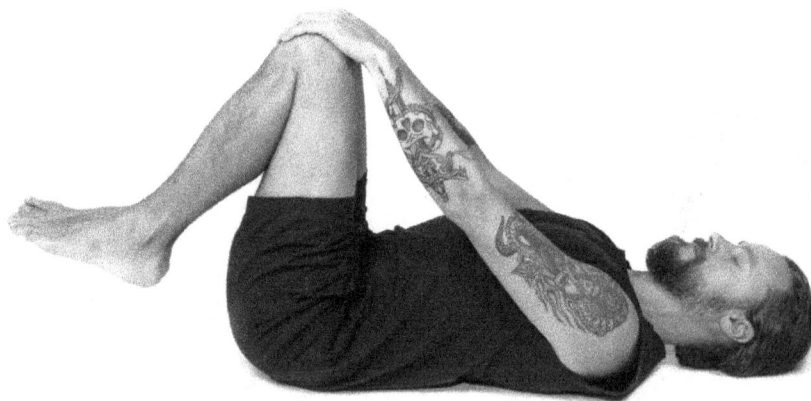

Getting there: Start by lying down on your back, knees toward your chest with hands resting on knees. This is the 'exhale' position.

Inhale as you move your knees away from your chest, keeping your feet relaxed and together.

<u>Extend your breath</u>: Count your breath silently, first establishing an even breath rhythm — inhale and exhale an equal count. Find a tempo that you can comfortably maintain for 5-10 breaths.

exhale

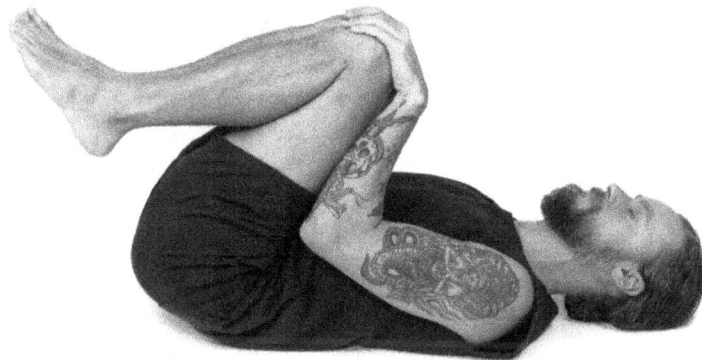

Exhale as you move your knees toward your chest. <u>Repeat</u> the movement a number of times. <u>Lengthen</u> just your exhalation by adding one count to each round. Keep your inhale the same length. <u>Benefit</u>: Lengthening your exhalation like this signals your nervous system to relax. Try this practice before bed or any time you would like to calm down.

4.0 flow sequences

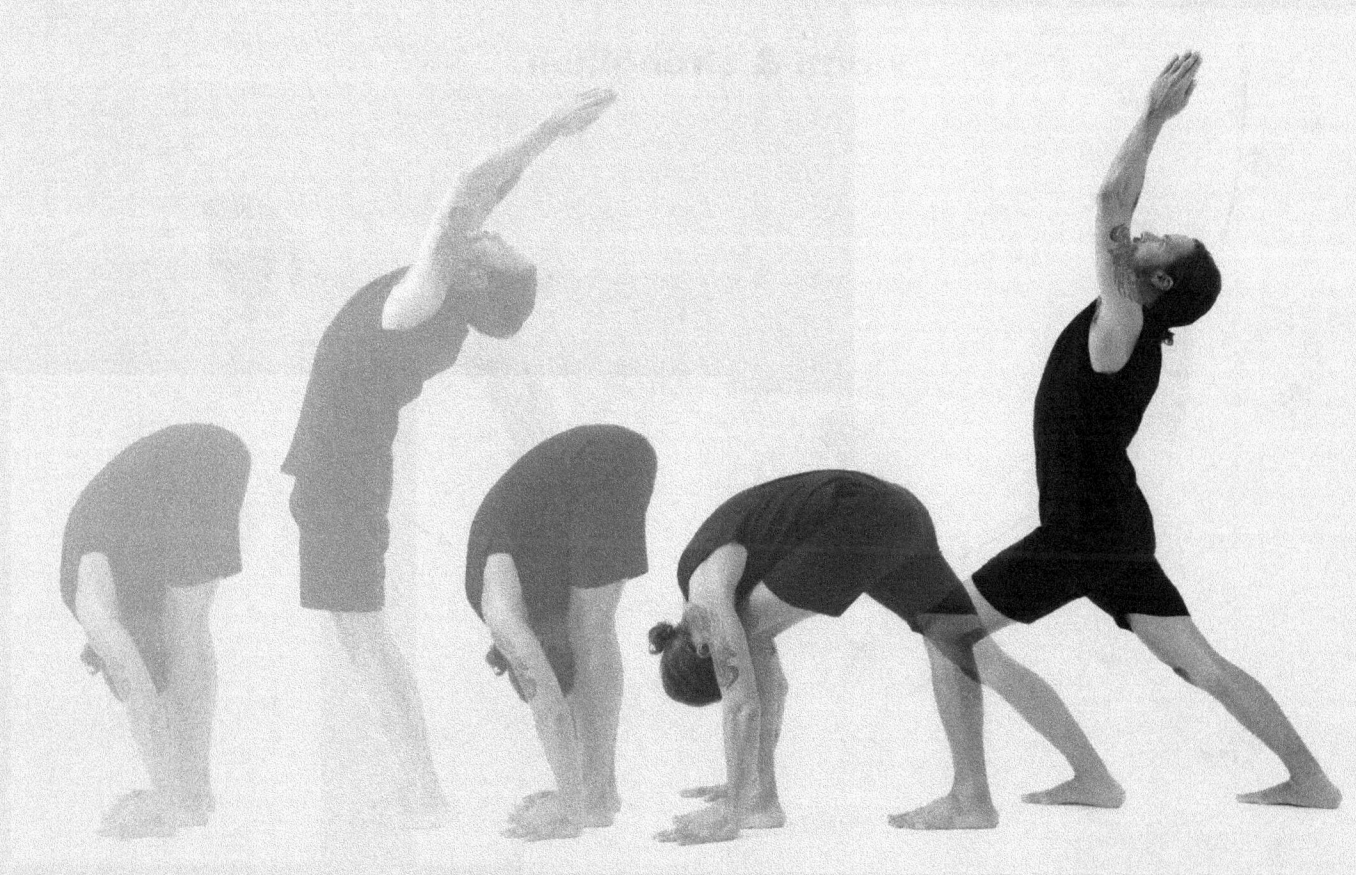

flow 4.1

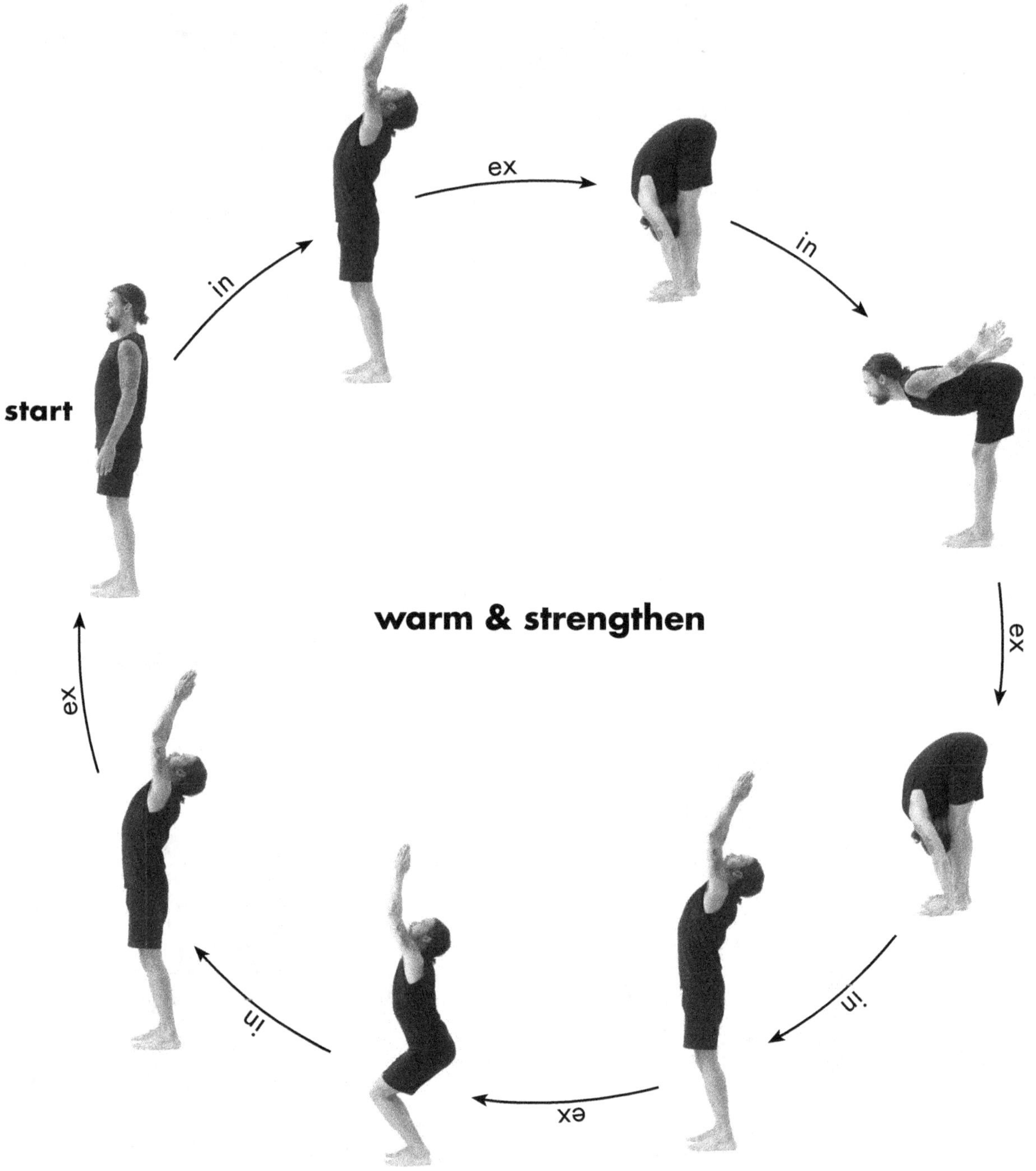

start

warm & strengthen

ex

in

in

ex

in

ex

in

ex

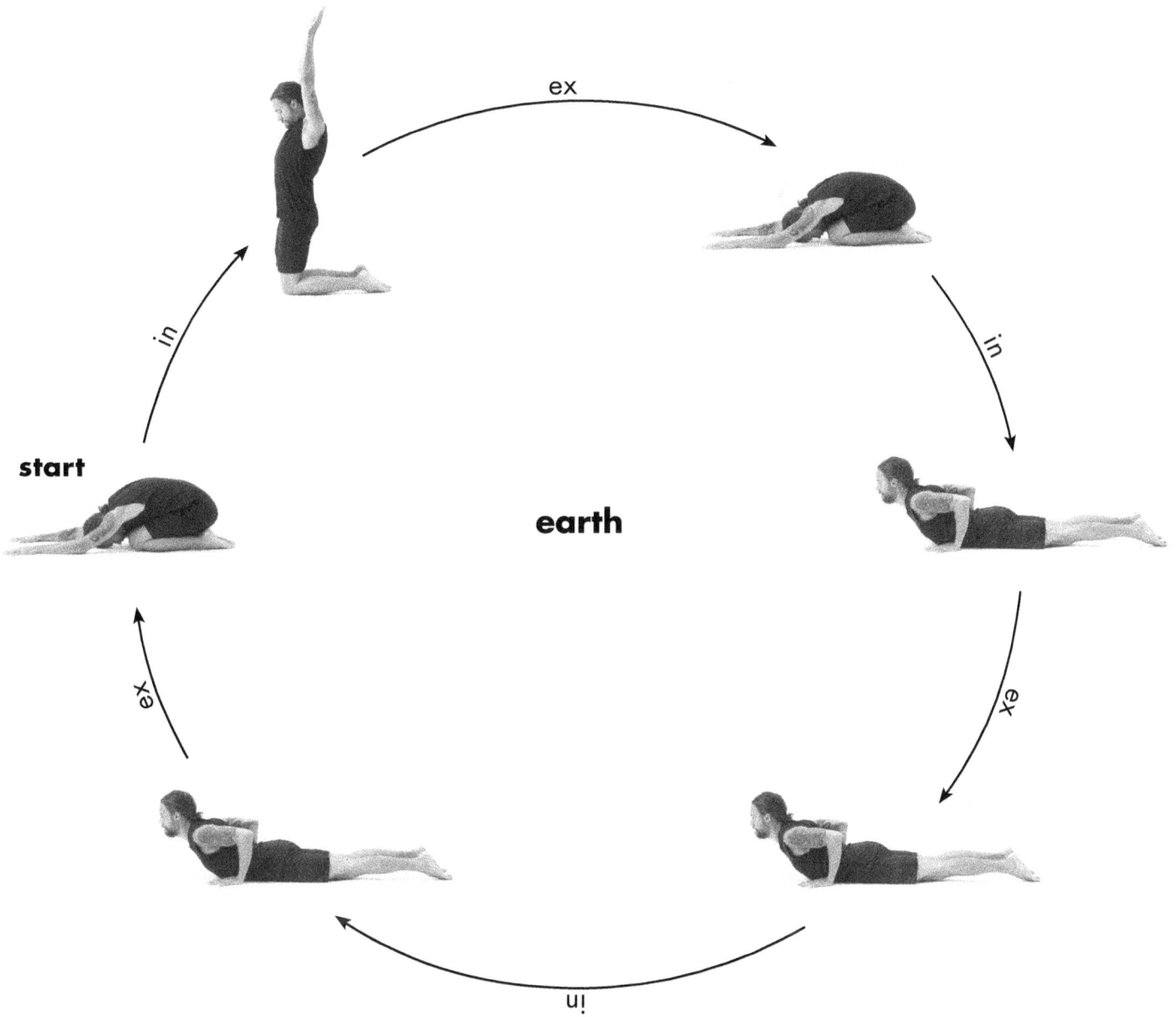

start

earth

ex

in

ex

in

in

ex

flow 4.3

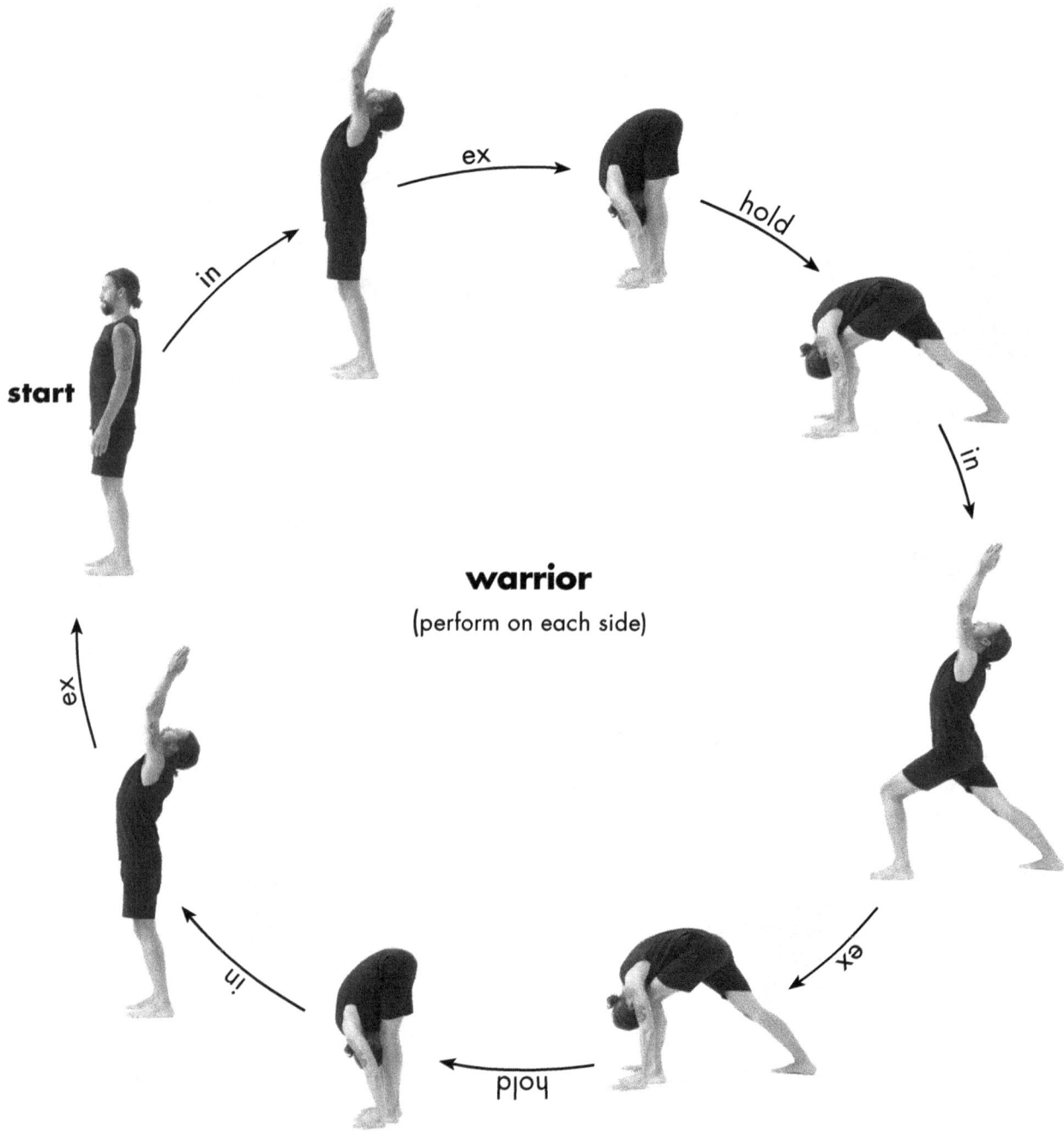

start

ex

in

hold

in

warrior

(perform on each side)

ex

hold

in

ex

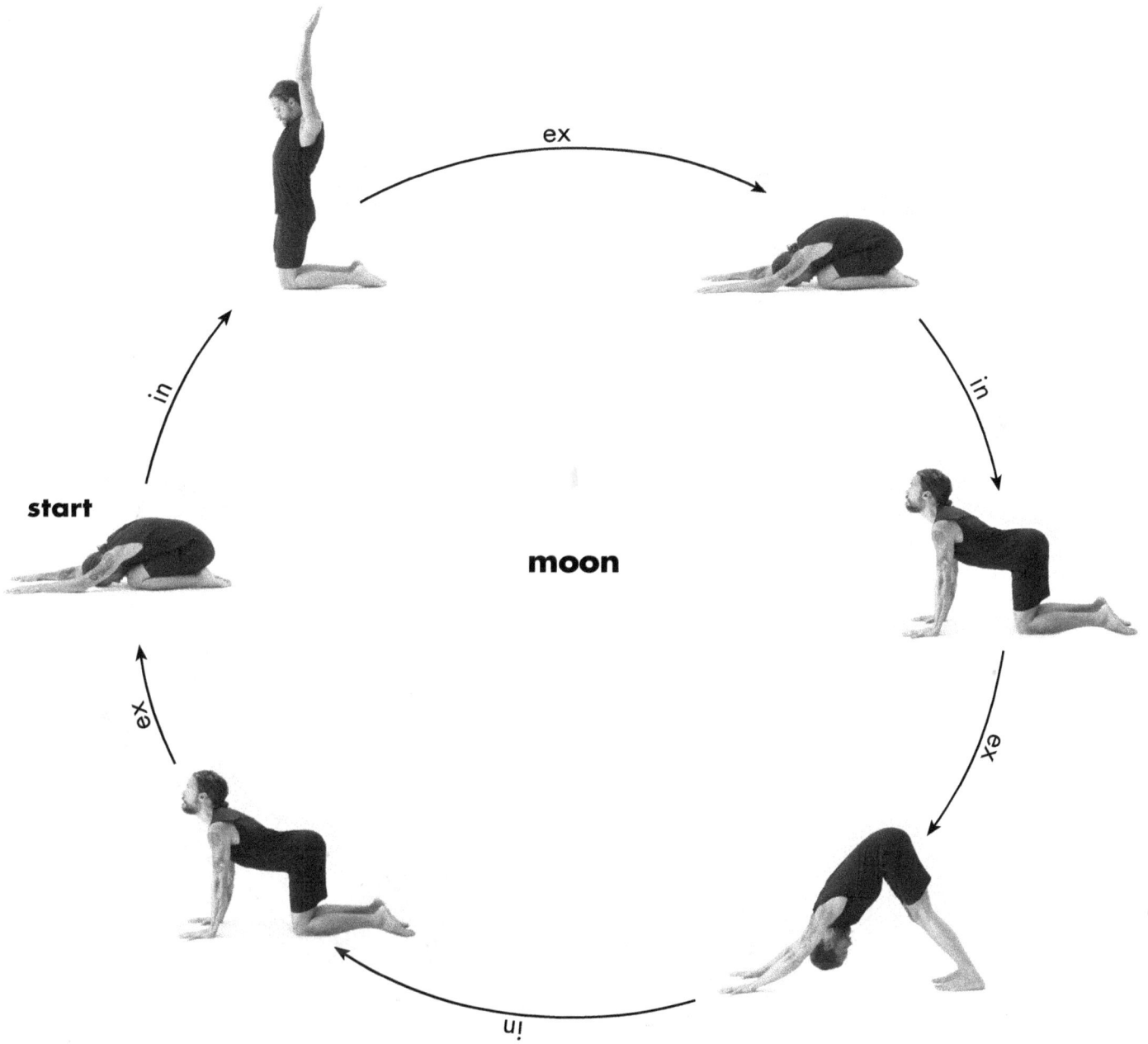

ex

in

start

in

moon

ex

in

ex

flow 4.5

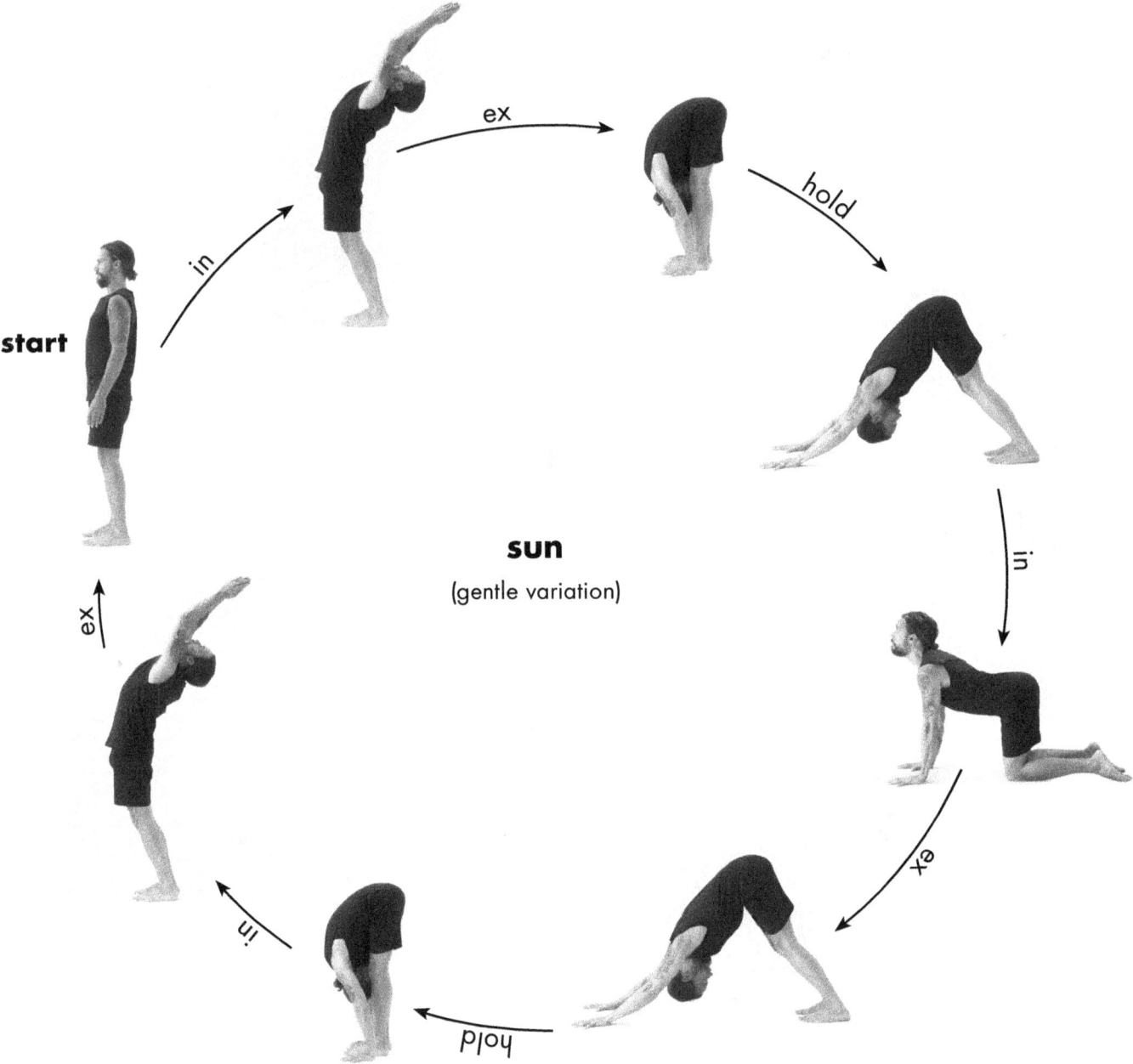

start

in

ex

hold

sun

(gentle variation)

in

ex

hold

in

ex

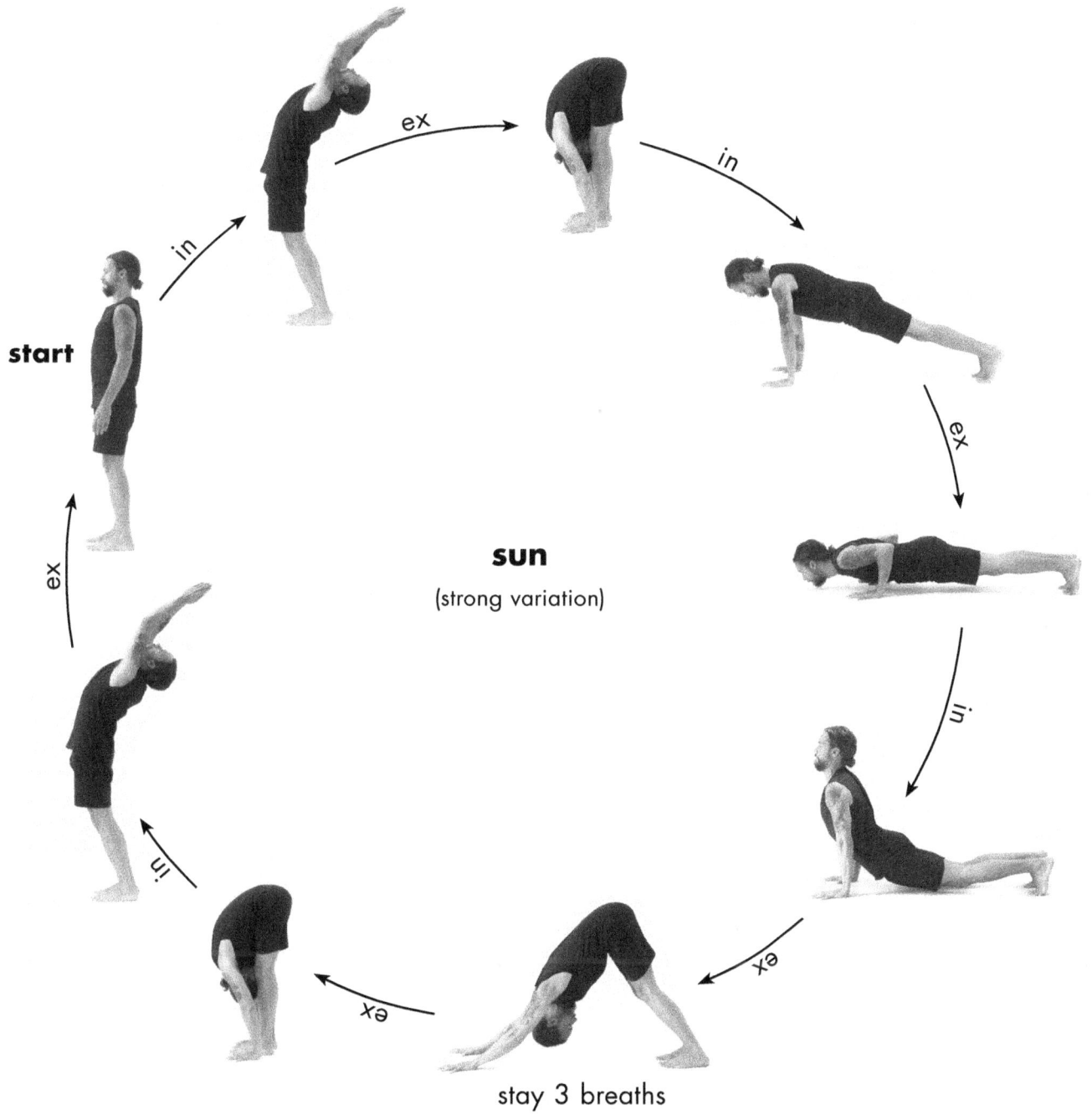

start

ex

in

in

ex

ex

in

stay 3 breaths

in

ex

sun

(strong variation)

5.0 practice

Put the Harmonic Movement method into practice.

A daily home practice is where you will really see the increasing long-term benefits of a consistent mindful movement practice, in both your body and your mind.

A regular practice that combines breath and mindful movement will help you maintain strength, balance and mobility, increase your energy levels, decrease stress and improve mental clarity.

The best way to establish a lasting daily practice is by keeping it simple at the outset and staying consistent for a significant, predetermined length of time. Even if you feel like you could manage a longer practice, try incorporating a short 10-20 minute sequence into your morning schedule for thirty days. After a full month of consistent practice your new healthy habit will be well-established and you can start adding to, or modifying the sequences in this section. *Keep it simple, be consistent* is your mantra.

sequence 5.1

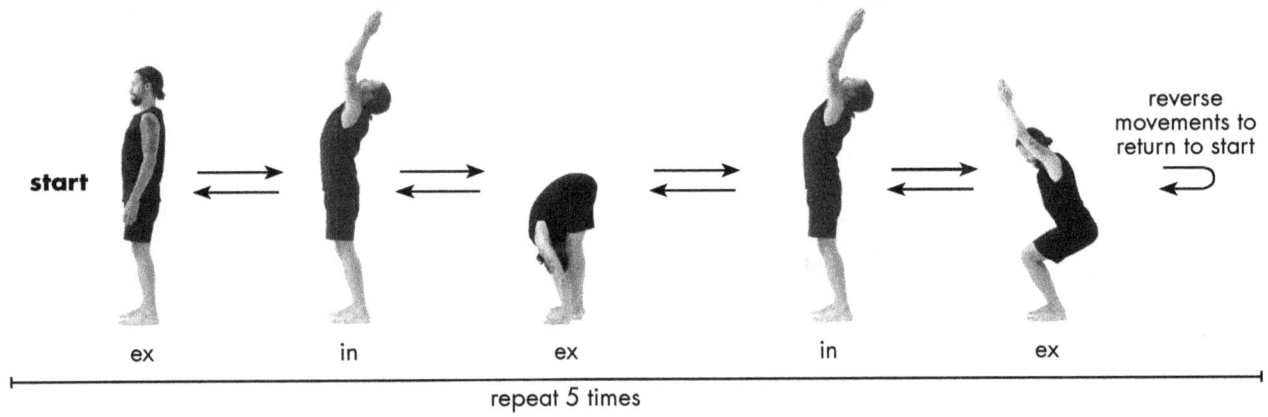

start   ex   in   ex   in   ex

reverse movements to return to start

repeat 5 times

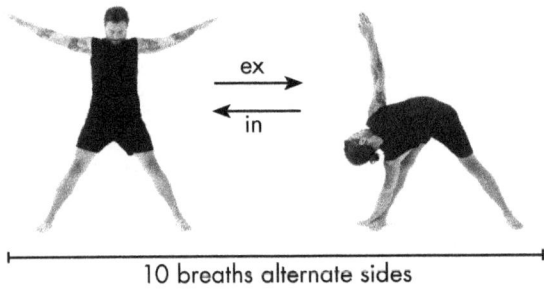

10 breaths alternate sides

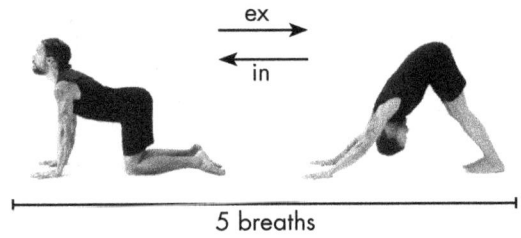

5 breaths

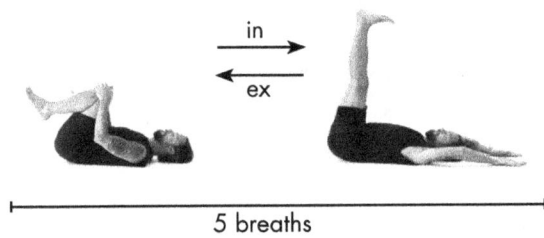

5 breaths

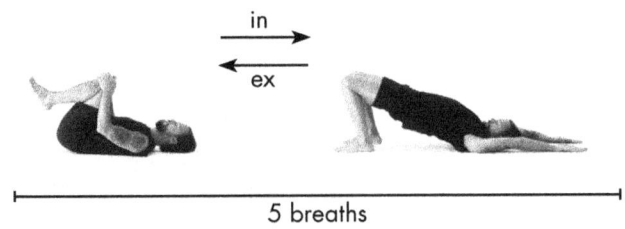

5 breaths

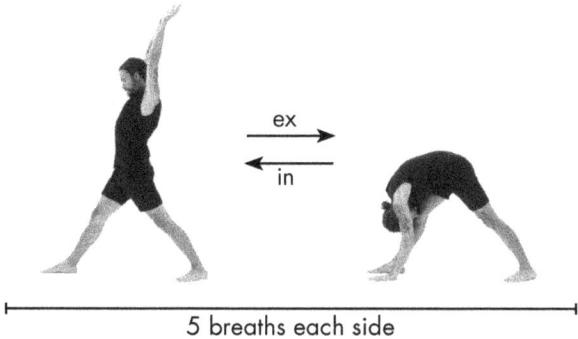

5 breaths each side

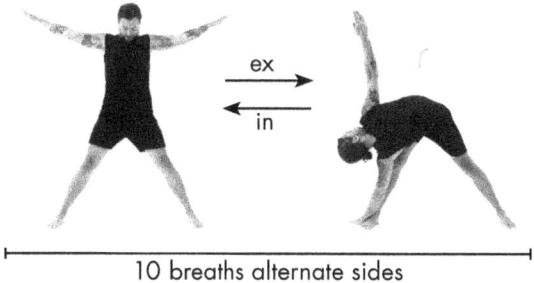

10 breaths alternate sides

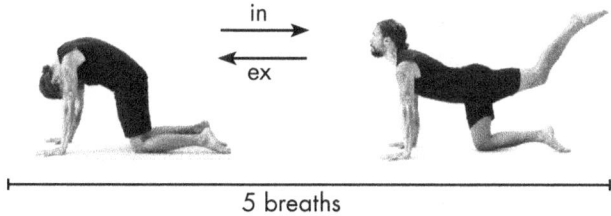

5 breaths

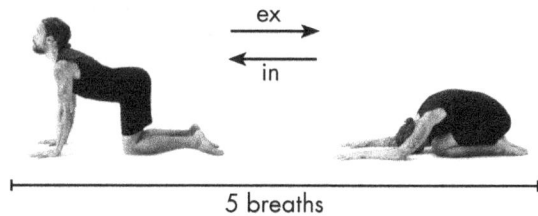

5 breaths

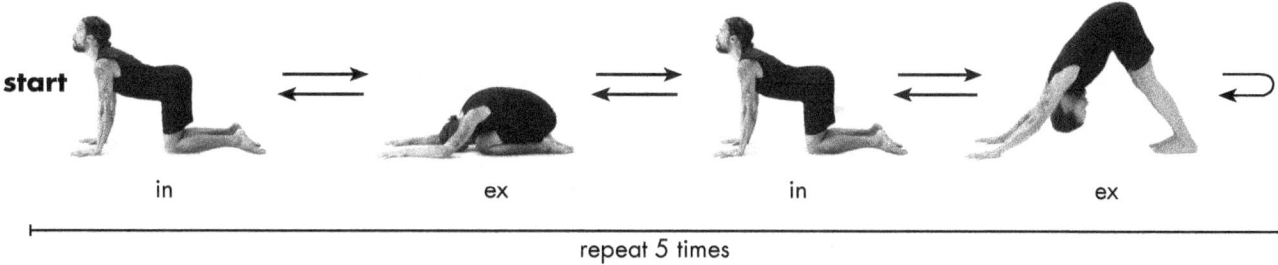

start

in   ex   in   ex

repeat 5 times

sequence 5.3

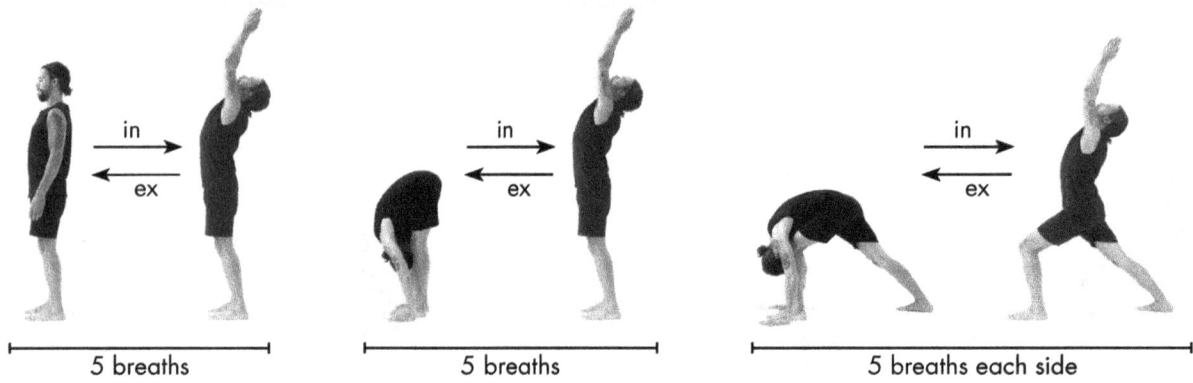

5 breaths	5 breaths	5 breaths each side

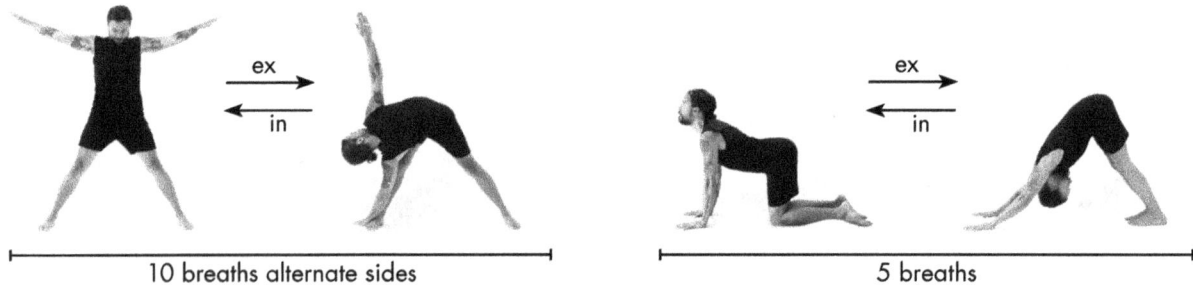

10 breaths alternate sides	5 breaths

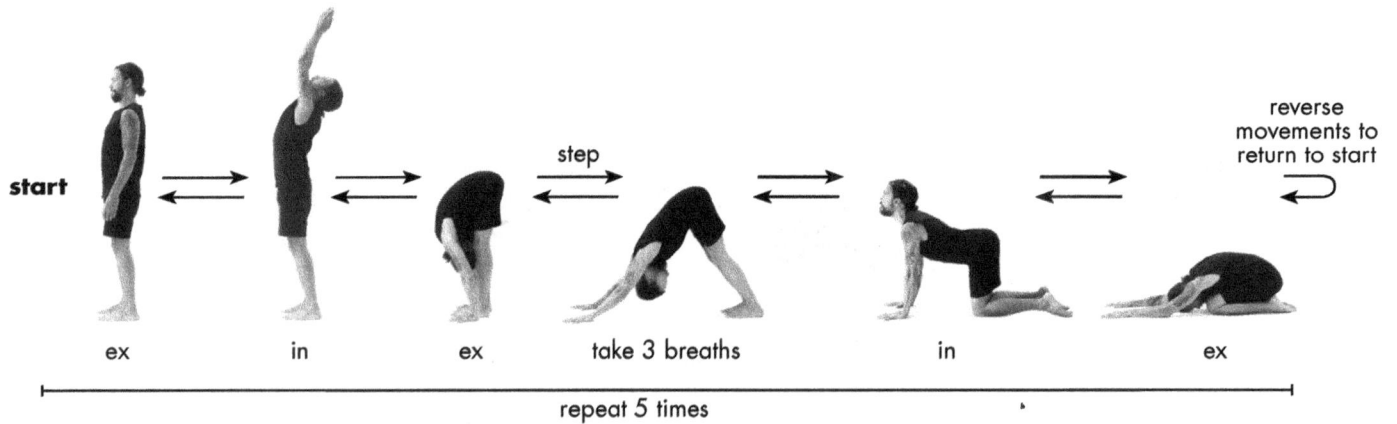

reverse movements to return to start

start   ex   in   ex   step   take 3 breaths   in   ex

repeat 5 times

ex →
← in

5 breaths each side

in →
← ex

5 breaths

ex →
← in

10 breaths alternate legs

ex →
← in

10 breaths alternate sides

rest

in →
← ex

10-20 breaths

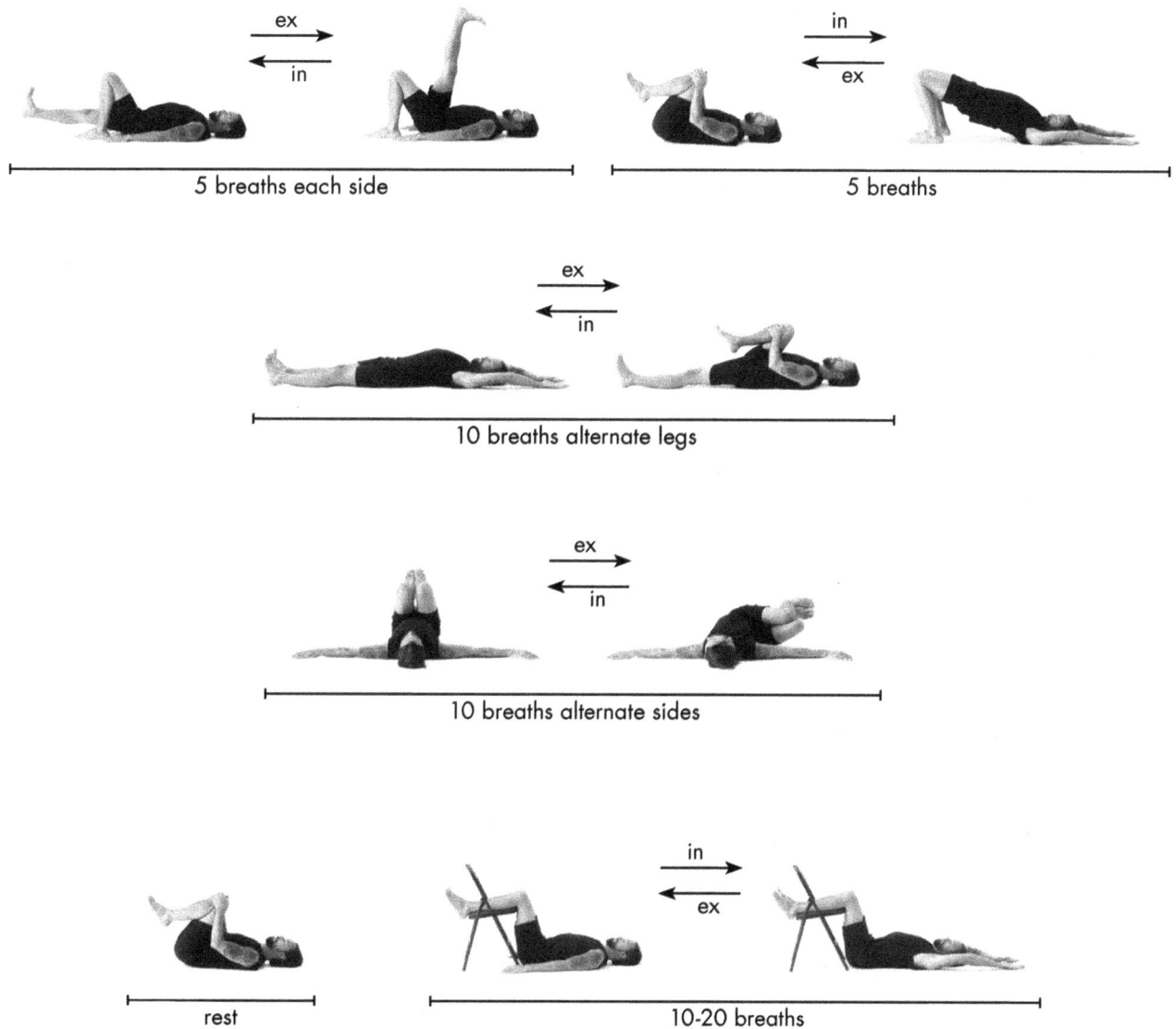

This sequence works as a complete restorative practice or
can be added on to sequence 5.2 or 5.3 to create a longer practice.

6.0 rest & reflect

Harmonic Movement creates the perfect conditions for a meditative state to arise naturally.

Allow 5-10 minutes after your movement practice to be still and observe the feeling in your body and the quality of your thoughts. You can do this as a formal seated meditation, or just lie down and rest. Don't try to force anything specific to happen — *just be.*

Following your meditation/rest period, you might feel inspired to write, draw, sing or play music. Harmonic Movement gets the creative juices flowing, so if inspiration happens, *express yourself!*

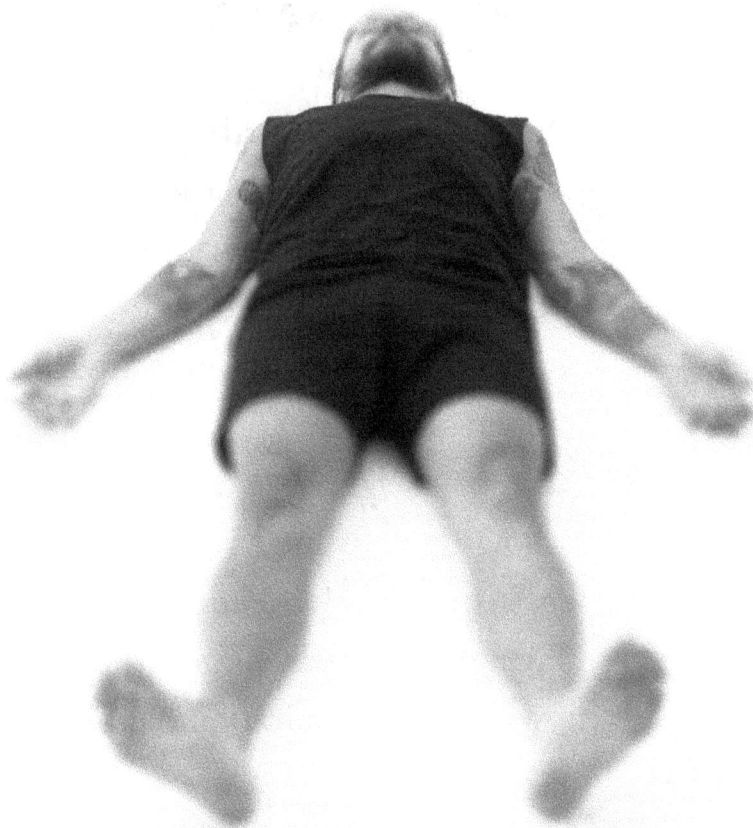

Lie down and let go. Arrange your body in a way that allows you to release all effort. Take some time and scan your body — imagine that you're drawing a map of your inner landscape. Allow your awareness to rest in the stillness of your whole body. Try to spend some time resting like this after every movement practice.

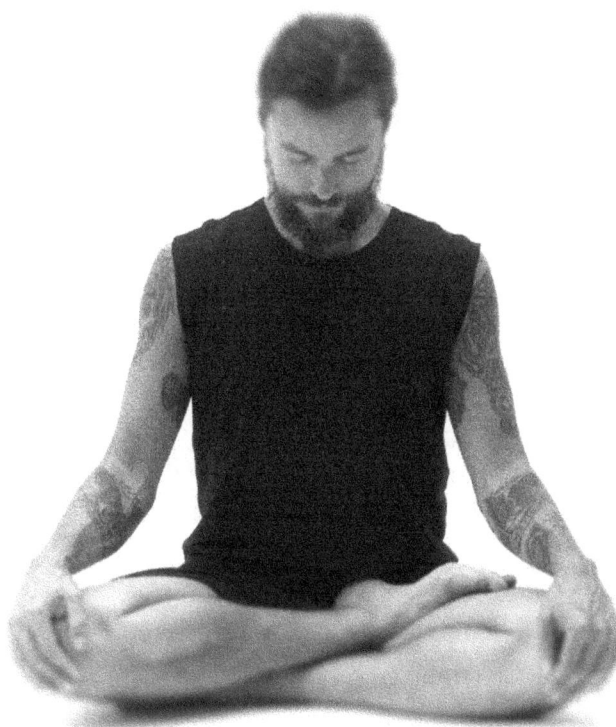

Quiet your mind. Listen to your body.

Sit in a position that is both stable and comfortable. Use a blanket or cushion under your hips
if needed. Close your eyes and quietly observe your breath, the sensations in your body and the
movement of your thoughts. Don't try to force anything to happen, just be.

07 create

The sequences in this book are only meant to provide you with a starting point for your practice.

Once you've practiced and mastered the Harmonic Movement method, you'll be able to infuse any movement with conscious breath, transforming it into a powerful moving meditation.

Fill the following pages with your own inspired flow sequences. To get you started, I've provided an example of how to sketch out sequences using stick figures and breath notation.

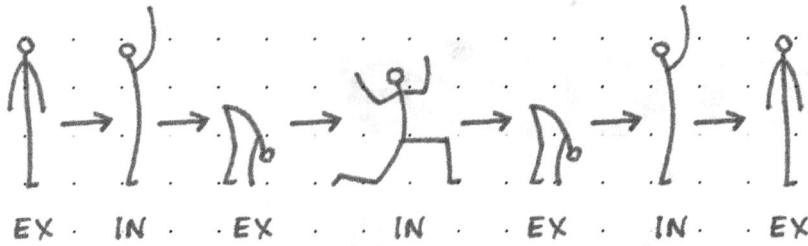 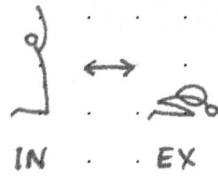

EX · IN · EX · IN · EX · IN · EX · · · IN · EX

168 create

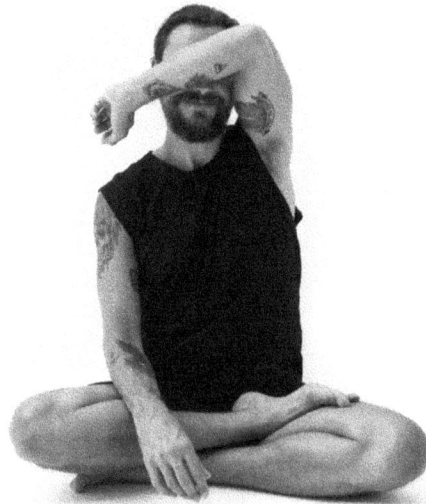

ABOUT THE AUTHOR

Brian James Kroeker has been studying and practicing
music, movement and creative arts for most of his life.
He teaches yoga and music in Montréal, Canada where he
lives with his wife Debbie and their two Boston Terriers,
Kingston and Sweetie.

www.ingramcontent.com/pod-product-compliance
Lightning Source LLC
Chambersburg PA
CBHW080359030426
42334CB00024B/2933